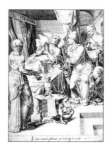

Bates D. Moses, MD
Board Certified Palliative Medicine
Co-Chair Bioethics Committee and Clinical Faculty Family
Medicine residency at Kaiser Permanente Riverside, CA
Clinical Preceptor, Biomedical Sciences,
University of California at Riverside, CA

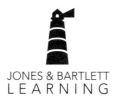

JONES & BARTLETT
LEARNING

World Headquarters
Jones & Bartlett Learning
5 Wall Street
Burlington, MA 01803
978-443-5000
info@jblearning.com
www.jblearning.com

Jones & Bartlett Learning books and products are available through most bookstores and online booksellers. To contact Jones & Bartlett Learning directly, call 800-832-0034, fax 978-443-8000, or visit our website, www.jblearning.com.

Production Credits
Sr. Acquisition Editor: Nancy Anastasi Duffy
Editorial Assistant: Marisa LaFleur
Production Assistant: Alex Schab
Marketing Manager: Rebecca Leitch
Manufacturing and Inventory Control Supervisor: Amy Bacus
Composition: CAE Solutions Corp.
Cover Design: Kristin Parker
Cover Image: Courtesy of The National Library of Medicine
Printing and Binding: Cenveo Publisher Services
Cover Printing: Cenveo Publisher Services

ISBN 13: 978-1-4496-3421-6

6048
Printed in the United States of America
16 15 14 13 12   10 9 8 7 6 5 4 3 2 1

PART 3: EMERGENCIES AND
FURTHER READING   121

11 Emergencies   123
    Actively Dying   123
    Acute Bleeding   124
    Anaphylaxis   126
    Cardiac Tamponade   126
    Cord Compression   127
    Hypercalcemia   128
    Increased Intracranial
      Pressure   129
    Serotonin Syndrome   130
    Superior Vena Cava
      Syndrome   131
    Tumor Lysis Syndrome   132
    Withdrawal Syndromes   133

12 Further Reading
    and References   135
    Background   135
    Communication   135
    Ethical Decision Making   136
    Prognostication   136
    Cultural and Religious
      Concerns   137
    Gastrointestinal and
      Genitourinary   137
    Neuropsychiatric   140
    Pain   142
    Respiratory   142
    Skin   143
    Emergencies   143

    Index   145

CONTENTS

Reviewers List | v
Note from the Author | vi
Acronyms | vii

PART 1: GOALS OF CARE | 1

1 **Background** | 3
Goals of Medicine | 3
Palliative Medicine | 3
U.S. 2010 Hospice
   Statistics | 8

2 **Communication** | 11
Palliative Care Teams | 11
The Patient | 13
Bad News | 16
The Family | 18

3 **Ethical Decision
Making** | 23
Ethical Principles | 23
Ethics Consultation | 24
Shared Decision Making | 27
Withholding Versus
   Withdrawing
   Treatment | 28
Death | 29
Physician-Assisted
   Suicide and Euthanasia | 30

4 **Prognostication** | 31
Basic Information | 31
Hospice Criteria | 31
Intensive Care Unit | 35
Disease Based Guidelines | 35

5 **Cultural and
Religious Concerns** | 39
Ethnic Views | 39
Spiritual Views | 41

PART 2: SYMPTOMS | 47

6 **Gastrointestinal
and Genitourinary** | 49
Anorexia-Cachexia
   Syndrome | 49
Ascites, Malignancy-
   Related | 52
Urinary Symptoms | 53
Abdominal Bloating
   and Gas | 55

Constipation and Bowel
   Obstruction | 56
Diarrhea | 59
Dyspepsia and
   Gastroesophageal
   Reflux Disease
   (GERD) | 61
Oropharynx: Dysphagia,
   Mucositis, Xerostomia,
   and Halitosis | 62
Nausea and Vomiting | 65

7 **Neuropsychiatric** | 69
Anxiety | 69
Delirium | 72
Grief and
   Bereavement | 75
Depression | 79
Fatigue | 83
Insomnia | 85

8 **Pain** | 87
Definitions | 87
Pain Descriptors | 87
Assessment | 88
Documenting Pain | 88
Management of Pain | 89
NSAIDs and
   Acetaminophen | 89
Opioids | 92
Adjuvants | 102
Procedures | 106
Radiopharmaceutical
   Therapies | 106
Specific Conditions | 107
Complementary
   Therapies | 108

9 **Respiratory** | 109
Chronic Cough | 109
Dyspnea | 110
Hiccups | 111
Oral Secretions | 112
Pleural Effusions | 113
Terminal Extubation
   Protocols | 114

10 **Skin** | 115
Malodorous Fungating
   Wounds | 115
Pressure Ulcers | 117
Pruritus | 118

REVIEWERS LIST

NOTE FROM THE AUTHOR

The *Tarascon Palliative Medicine Pocketbook* is intended to be a quick "in the field" or "just in time" guide. I hope that most members of palliative care teams or the many other professionals also helping suffering patients can find something helpful in this pocket reference. If you find an error or wish to make a suggestion please let us know.

I would like to thank my many wonderful mentors during my medical career (Dr. Cao, Dr. McDonald, Dr. Gebreselassie, Dr. Cuyegkeng, Dr. Lewis, and many many more) and my colleagues in palliative care (Anna, Pia, Kristen, and more). Thank-you to all the experts and researchers in the field who are advancing the field and many whose findings or recommendations are summarized in the book. Thank-you also to the publishing team who helped put this all together and to those who've reviewed portions of this book.

This book is dedicated to my wife Kristen, my daughters Claire and Jasmine, my parents Devadas and Dharmaseeli, my sister Ranjini, and grandparents "Patti" and "Thatha." My daughter's reminded me that when a choice comes between playing with them or researching and writing a book, what I initially thought was an easy choice (kids first!), in practice wasn't. So to all healthcare professionals who also take their work home with them, remember that taking care of yourself and your family will help you take better care of your patients.

Bates D. Moses, MD

ACRONYMS

ABG	arterial blood gas
ACE	angiotensin-converting enzyme
ADLs	activities of daily living
ALS	amyotrophic lateral sclerosis
CAD	coronary artery disease
CBC	complete blood count
CNS	central nervous system
COPD	chronic obstructive pulmonary disease
CPAP	continuous positive airway pressure
CPR	cardiopulmonary resuscitation
CrCl	creatinine clearance
CSF	cerebrospinal fluid
DIC	disseminated intravascular coagulation
DIIA	docosahexaenoic acid
DSM-IV	*Diagnostic and Statistical Manual of Mental Disorders 4th ed.*
DSM-V	*Diagnostic and Statistical Manual of Mental Disorders 5th ed.*
ECOG	Eastern Cooperative Oncology Group
ED	emergency department
EGD	esophagogastroduodenoscopy
EPA	eicosapentaenoic acid
ESR	erythrocyte sedimentation rate
ESRD	end-stage renal disease
ER	extended release
ET tube	endotracheal tube
FEV1	forced expiratory volume in 1 second
GAD	generalized anxiety disorder
GERD	gastroesophageal reflux disease
GFR	glomerular filtration rate
GI	gastrointestinal
GU	genitourinary
HR	heart rate
HSV	herpes simplex virus
HTN	hypertension
IBS	irritable bowel syndrome
ICP	intracranial pressure
ICU	intensive care unit
IM	intramuscular
INR	international normalized ratio
IR	immediate release
IV	intravenous
IVFs	intravenous fluids
KS	Kaposi's sarcoma
MAC infection	Mycobacterium avium-intracellulare
MAOI	monoamine oxidase inhibitor

MRC	Medical Research Council
MS	multiple sclerosis
NMDA	N-Methyl-D-aspartate glutamate receptor
NS	normal saline
NSAIDs	nonsteroidal anti-inflammatory drugs
NYHA	New York Heart Association
PCA	patient controlled analgesia
PEG	percutaneous endoscopic gastrostomy
PEEP	positive-end expiratory pressure
PO	by mouth/orally
POLST/MOLST/ POST/MOST	physician or medical orders for life sustaining treatment/physician or medical orders for scope of treatment
PR	by rectum
prn	as needed
ODT	orally disintegrating tab
q	every
qAM	in the morning
qPM	in the evening
q hs	at bedtime
RMM	respirations by mandibular movement
SAAG	serum ascites albumin gradient
SBP	systolic blood pressure
SL	sublingual
SNRI	serotonin–norepinephrine reuptake inhibitor
SQ	subcutaneous
SR	sustained release
SSRI	selective serotonin reuptake inhibitors
TCA	tricyclic antidepressant
TIPS	transjugular intrahepatic portosystemic shunt
TPN	total parenteral nutrition
UGI	upper gastrointestinal
UTI	urinary tract infection
VC	vital capacity
VEGF	vascular endothelial growth factor
WBC	white blood cell count
WHO	World Health Organization

PART I: GOALS OF CARE

1 ■ BACKGROUND

GOALS OF MEDICINE

I. **Goals of medicine: to cure, to care, to comfort**
   A. To cure: curative medicine's aim is to avoid a premature death. The physician should be skilled in diagnosing and treating curable conditions.
   B. To care: to improve health and avoid a premature death while respecting the patient as a person.
   C. To comfort: to relieve suffering and help with options when cure is not possible.
   D. Nole that the preservation of life alone cannot be a primary goal for medicine.
      1. All humans die, so this goal is unattainable unless reframed as attempting to avoid a premature death (i.e., if the condition can be cured or maintained as long as possible as a chronic condition).
      2. Most physicians are trained during medical school and residency to view death as a failure. Weekly conferences ask what was missed or done wrong, implying that if everything is done correctly patients would not die.
      3. National statistics monitor mortality rates and attempt to identify "preventable" deaths based on best available metrics, but the human mortality rate remains at 100% and changing the location of death may or may not mean improved quality.
      4. These endeavors improve the quality of medicine and typically improve quantity and quality of lives by minimizing premature deaths. However, these same interventions may make it difficult to acknowledge when patients are truly suffering or when patients are dying.

PALLIATIVE MEDICINE

I. **Palliative care**
   A. Model for quality, compassionate care.
   B. Goal is to prevent and relieve suffering by early identification and impeccable assessment and treatment of suffering in patients with life-limiting conditions. Hospice can be conceptualized as the last 6 months of palliative care.

    C. Principles
        1. Primary: team-based approach involving collaborative and collegial model of shared decision-making that should be incorporated into healthcare systems and practiced by all healthcare professionals. It does not need to be called *palliative care* as its principles can be implemented throughout the healthcare system for patients with any type of illness, especially serious illnesses.
        2. Secondary: specialty-level services that are provided by certified palliative medicine professionals. Physician members of palliative care teams have subspecialty-level board certification in hospice and palliative medicine who can provide consultative services (clinic-based, home-based, or hospital-based) or primary services (such as in a hospital palliative care unit) and work closely with other certified palliative care team members (nurse practitioners, physician assistants, nurses, social workers, chaplains, and pharmacists). Patients needing referral to (or being seen by) a specialty palliative service should have a serious illness with identified or anticipated difficult-to-control symptoms (physical, mental, or social).
        3. Palliative care principles can be provided concurrently with curative, restorative, or preventive medicine. It can be provided everywhere that a patient may be treated (ambulatory settings, homebound patients, skilled nursing home patients, hospitalized patients, emergency room patients).

II. Hospice

    A. Subset of palliative care.
    B. Covered by Medicare and most commercial insurance as a benefit for patients whose life expectancy is less than 6 months, assuming the disease's "natural" course.
       • Code status, automated implanted cardiac defibrillators, and other similar situations cannot be used to determine eligibility.
    C. Primary goal is quality of life and symptom control (comfort).
    D. Provided where patients live (in the community, such as a home, board and care, or custodial nursing home facility).
    E. Patients can revoke hospice at any time.
    F. Provider can discharge a patient if found to have improving prognosis:
        1. For example, a patient may have been on a liver transplant list and a liver has been found.
        2. Cannot discharge a patient if admitted to the hospital solely for refractory symptom control.
    G. Initially certified by two physicians for two 90-day periods (6 months) and then renewed as needed in 60-day intervals.

TABLE 1.1 Basic Hospice Services

Core	Noncore
Nursing	Therapists (physical, occupational, speech)
Physician	Hospice home aides
Counseling (at least 1 year of bereavement, dietary, and spiritual)	Registered dietitians
Social services	Volunteers (which should be >5% of total care)

Source: Data from http://www.cms.gov/Hospice/

III. **Core and noncore services**
   A. Most interventions are covered if the primary intent is palliation
      1. Must document the symptom being palliated.
      2. Includes medications, supplies, equipment, labs, diagnostic tests, palliative treatments (radiation, chemotherapy, thoracentesis, paracentesis, surgery), enteral products (head and neck cancer patients with PEG), and TPN (if no functional GI tract).
IV. **Whole person care**
   A. Integral part of hospice and palliative care.
   B. Goal is to focus on whole person symptom management, not hasten or postpone death.
      • Symptom management often inadvertently prolongs life.
   C. Helps patients live as actively as possible.
   D. Treats the whole family, as defined by the patient.
      • Includes bereavement care for family members.
   E. Treatments that improve quality of life are pursued.
   F. ED visits.
      1. Hospice is a destination program; palliative care is not.
      2. Palliative care is often provided concurrently with traditional care with curative or maintenance intent.
         a. It is not an "either/or," but a "both/and" model.
         b. Seamless integration is becoming the standard of care.
      3. Regardless of support program, the patient or surrogate felt concerned that whatever the issue was, it could not be taken care of in the prior setting.
      4. Possible reasons for ED visits include: concerns due to difficulty coping with impending loss of life (leading to requests for previously discontinued or uninitiated interventions), poor symptom control, malfunction of current support devices, or delays (real or perceived) in home team response to crisis scenarios.

5. When a hospice patient arrives in the ED, immediately notify the hospice staff after the trigger for the visit has been identified.
   a. Immediately obtain social services and chaplain consultation for patient and family support; help identify surrogates and locate advance directives.
   b. Simultaneously treat distressing symptoms.
   c. If rapid deterioration is noted, make a clear recommendation based on the patient's known values and reality of the current medical situation.
      i. Depending on discussion and plan of care, formally consult hospice (if admission not required or unclear) and/or palliative medicine (if admission appears to be required) and other specialists as appropriate to the situation.
      ii. At times, hospital-level care is needed for difficult symptom control.
         (A) If an inpatient hospice facility or inpatient palliative care unit is not available, the emergency room and hospital become the safety net for dying patients with distressing and difficult-to-control symptoms.
6. The most common diagnosis codes (in descending order) for ED visits during the last 6 months of life and last 2 weeks of life are listed in **Table 1.2.**

TABLE 1.2 Terminal Patient's ED Visit Diagnosis Reasons

	ED Visits Within 6 Months of Death	ED Visits Within 2 Weeks of Death
1	Abdominal pain	Lung cancer
2	Lung cancer	Dyspnea
3	Pneumonia	Pneumonia
4	Dyspnea	Abdominal pain
5	Malaise and fatigue	Malaise and fatigue
6	Chest pain	Palliative care (on a palliative service)
7	Pleural effusion	Dehydration
8	Nausea or vomiting	Pleural effusion
9	Anemia	Altered consciousness
10	Back pain	Pancreatic cancer
11	Constipation	Colon cancer
12	Fever	Heart failure
13	Dehydration	Intestinal obstruction
14	Chronic obstructive pulmonary disease	Breast cancer
15	Urinary tract infection	Gastrointestinal hemorrhage

Source: Adapted from Barbera, L., Taylor, C., & Dudgeon, D. (2010). Why do patients with cancer visit the emergency department near the end of life? *Canadian Medical Association Journal*, 182(6), 563–568.

I. Pediatrics and palliative care

A. Differences compared to adult and geriatric palliative care
- Causes of death
  a. Infant mortality (younger than 1 year old): usually due to congenital disorders, SIDS, or prematurity.
  b. Children (1–14 years old): primarily due to unintentional injuries (trauma due to motor vehicle accidents, homicide, suicide, and drowning), then cancers (though majority can be put into remission), then cardiac etiologies, and finally congenital diseases.
  c. Teenagers and young adults (15–24 years old): also due to unintentional injuries (with higher rates of homicide and suicide than younger children), then cancer.

B. Pediatric palliative care
1. Consider reframing as "supportive care" due to high remission rates for many childhood cancers, and this wording seems more acceptable to family.
2. Emphasis is on optimal living and should coincide with restorative care and treatments.
3. It is best to initiate palliative support when a life-threatening condition is diagnosed (even prenatally) to provide long-term support and assist in minimizing distressing symptoms.

C. Children's view of death
1. Finalism: Children believe that bad things only happen to bad people.
   a. If they feel pain, they may not admit to it to avoid admitting to "being bad."
2. Ask older children questions to understand their inner thoughts better:
   a. For example, if they ask "Am I dying?" or "What happens after you die?" try to find out why the question is entering their mind (as appropriate for their age) and first clarify the emotion behind the question.
   b. If the child is using concrete language, then answers should also be in concrete language.

D. Parental support
- This is crucial as a child's illness can devastate a marriage; initiate couples' therapy early and provide community support resources for the entire family.

TABLE 1.3 Children's Views of Death

Age (years)	View of Death and Worries	Interventions
0–2	Death is separation from family.	Touch, hold, skin contact.
2–6	Death is a sleep state (i.e., reversible). The child worries about eating, breathing, jumping. Death is from being "bad."	Provide concrete interventions as appropriate to help with such responses as child's lack of appetite/refusal to eat. Tell child it's not a result of being bad.
6–8	Death is irreversible but unpredictable. The child fears abandonment and loss of control.	Emphasize presence and availability. Interventions should maximize child's sense of control.
>8	Death is irreversible and universal.	Allow anger; provide peer support and counseling.

Source: Data from Himebauch A, Arnold R, May C. Grief in Children and Developmental Concepts of Death. Fast Facts and Concepts. June 2005; 138. Available at: http://www.eperc.mcw.edu/EPERC/FastFactsIndex/ff_138.htm

U.S. 2010 HOSPICE STATISTICS

I. **Summary**
   A. The trend is that an increasing number of deaths in the United States occur with patients receiving hospice services. In 2010 41.9% of all deaths occurred under hospice care.
      • Just over 1 million out of nearly 2.5 million deaths.
   B. 16% of hospice patients discharged or self-revoked from hospice mainly due to extended prognosis or re-initiating curative treatment as primary goal.
   C. 35.3% died or were discharged within 7 days of admission to hospice, 27.0% within 8–29 days, 17.2% within 30–89 days, 8.7% within 90–179 days, and 11.8% 180 days or longer.
      • Median length of service was 19.7 days.
II. **Location**
   A. 66.7% of hospice patients died primarily at their residence (home, residential facility, or nursing home).
   B. 21.9% of hospice patients died in a hospice inpatient facility.
   C. 11.4% of hospice care patients died in an acute care hospital.

III. **Demographics**
   A. 56% of hospice patients were female.
   B. 82.7% were age 65 or older (<0.5% were pediatric population).
   C. Caucasians made up 77.3%, followed by multiracial (11%), African American (8.9%), Asian/Pacific Islander (2.5%), and Native American Indian (0.3%).

IV. **Diagnosis**
   A. Top 5 diagnoses of hospice patients
      1. Cancer: 35.6%
      2. Heart disease: 14.3%
      3. Dementia: 13%
      4. Unspecified: 13%
      5. Lung disease: 8.3%

2 ■ COMMUNICATION

PALLIATIVE CARE TEAMS

I. **Team model and composition**
   A. Primarily utilize the interdisciplinary or transdisciplinary team model.
   B. Medicare requires 4 core members (physician, nurse, social services, and spiritual counselor).
      1. Physician: responsible for overall medical care, provides certifying diagnosis and prognostication information.
      2. Nurse: acts as the patient care coordinator, completing assessments and implementing interventions.
      3. Social services: offers basic counseling and community assistance.
      4. Spiritual counselor: offers spiritual assessment and access to spiritual care.
      5. Other team members:
         a. Volunteers: offer companionship, help with chores and errands (cooking, housework, yard work).
         b. Patient and family can be considered team members.
         c. No leader is specified, however most patients and surrogates look to the physician as the de facto leader during family meetings and for treatment recommendations.

II. **Collaborative team development**
   A. Four phases
      1. Forming
         a. Team members are guarded, sizing up and eventually testing each other; they desire to be accepted by the team and avoid conflict.
      2. Storming
         a. There is increasing defensiveness and frustrations, but natural leaders begin to emerge. This is a normal and healthy part of team development, but some teams may get stuck in this stage.
      3. Norming
         a. Common goals are identified, roles become clarified; all team members take responsibility for the team's success.
      4. Performing
         a. Team members function as a unit and without the need for external supervision. Supervisors of these teams almost always act as team members. These teams may revert to prior phases as team members or supervisors change.

B. Effective teams have the following in common:
1. Clear goals (identifying clear problems to be solved)
2. Are results driven (have clear, measurable, time-limited objectives)
3. Competent members
4. Committed members
5. Principled leadership
6. Strong institutional support

C. Team conflicts are typically due to:
1. Relationship conflicts (personality issues)
   a. Be positive and proactive, and identify and separate the problem from the personality. Teach all team members basic conflict resolution skills.
2. Task conflicts (disagreements on work responsibilities)
   a. Roles need to be clarified.
3. Process conflicts (disagreements on strategies pursued)
   a. Proactively practice open communication while maintaining commitment to the patient's goals.

D. Burnout
1. Take care of yourself and your team. You cannot maximize care for your patients if your needs are not being met. If you notice in yourself or team members some or all of the following, it is time to seek help.
   a. Stress arousal: anxiety, irritability, hypertension, bruxism, insomnia, palpitations, forgetfulness, headaches
   b. Energy conservation: work tardiness, procrastination, resentment, morning fatigue, social withdrawal, increased alcohol or caffeine consumption, apathy
   c. Exhaustion: chronic sadness, depression, chronic heartburn, diarrhea, constipation, chronic mental and physical fatigue, desire to drop out of society
   d. Other signs:
      i. Overconscientious, increasing preoccupation with patients and/or frequent checking in after normal work hours
      ii. Loss of sense of humor
      iii. Increasing conflicts with staff, team members, or patients
      iv. Increasing difficulties at home
      v. Sense of helplessness
      vi. Increasing errors of judgment and difficulty concentrating
      vii. Addictive behaviors (drugs, gambling)
2. Burnout-reduction techniques
   a. Self-care basics (nutrition, exercise, sunshine, rest and relationships — spiritual and personal); recognize you are doing the best you can with limited resources
   b. Obtain counseling (do not self-prescribe medication)
   c. Debrief with a trusted team member or supervisor
   d. Last resort: job change (temporary or permanent)

THE PATIENT

I. **Communication basics**
   A. Talk is not enough.
      - Empathic listening and silence should take priority.
   B. Patients can sense your withdrawal, so remember to stay in contact despite difficulty with managing the disease or with patient's or family's understanding of the disease.
      1. Honor a patient's need for some level of denial.
      2. Don't focus only on the disease, focus also on the impact on their personal lives.
   C. Communication elements
      1. Understanding
         a. Find out how much the patient wants to know and who they want you to share information with.
         b. Until a patient/surrogate feels understood as a person, it is unlikely that they can think clearly about decisions that need to be made.
      2. Transmitting information
         a. Frequently pause and check for understanding.
      3. Decision making
         a. Create a dialogue with patient and family, exploring concerns and options.
         b. Reluctance for decision-making can be both patient/surrogate based and provider based
            i. Initiating discussions early allows for more informed decision making later.
            ii. Poor communication early results in ethical and legal issues later.
            iii. Subtle, nonverbal cues from physicians inform patients that such discussions are unwelcome, uncomfortable, or just not needed at this time.
   D. Barriers
      1. The need to initially deny/ignore life-threatening conditions
      2. The need to protect/preserve themselves and/or their family
      3. The physicians need to protect themselves from seeing what is happening
      4. Fear of death and dying
      5. Physician and other provider barriers
         a. Fear of being changed
            i. Providers rarely emerge unaffected by these life-changing events.
         b. Fear of expressing or eliciting emotions
         c. Fear of psychologically harming patient
      6. Patient barriers
         a. Distressing physical symptoms have not yet been controlled (obtain palliative specialty help early)

    b. Expectations on the current state of medicine
    c. Cultural differences
  7. Vocabulary barriers
    a. Using medical terminology interchangeably with layperson terminology
      i. For example, eating means chewing and swallowing, feeding means spooning food into someone else's mouth.
      ii. Define and use the proper terms of nasogastric or gastrostomy tube (or parenteral nutrition) for providing artificial nutrition. Consider utilizing drawings or videos to improve patient literacy and understanding.
      iii. Realize some artificial means of providing nutrition have become so common and assumed (such as bottle-feeding an infant) that the term *artificial* has lost its meaning to many. This does not mean that an accurate informed consent should not still take place.

TABLE 2.1 Empathic Strategies for Patient Interaction

Nonverbal Tips	Verbal Tips

• Sitting
  ○ At or below patient's eye level.
  ○ Sit as close as appropriate (2–3 feet).
  ○ Sit in a relaxed position with a slight lean toward the patient.
  ○ If possible sit in a circle, consider without a table barrier, consider mixed in among family members.
• Limit healthcare team members—patients and surrogates should outnumber the number of healthcare professionals participating otherwise may inadvertently portray a sense of power and authority by the health care team.
• Avoid invading others personal space (such as a bed without invitation).
• Avoid squatting (appears you are in a hurry).
• Caution with sustained eye contact (such as with some Asian, African, or American Indian cultures).
	• Observe for patient's nonverbal cues ("As we talked I noticed your eyes filled with tears, tell me more about what you're feeling or thinking about right now?").
	• Actively listen by acknowledging, clarifying, reassuring, and validating patient's emotions.
	  ○ By first identifying and responding to the emotion behind a patient's or family member's statements you demonstrate empathy by acknowledging your patient as a person.
	• Ask open-ended questions ("Tell me about…").
	  ○ Attempt to understand your patient from your patient's point of view.
	• Encourage to keep speaking ("uh-hum," "hmm," "oh," "and?," "then?," "is there anything else you would like to add before we move on?").
	• Repeat, paraphrase, reflect, and clarify what a patient has said to confirm understanding.
	• Use therapeutic humor carefully. When used appropriately you may be the only person a patient can safely share humor with.

II. Goal setting
A. Relationship building
1. Develop a relationship with the patient. ("Tell me about yourself.")
2. Keep discussions patient centered, not disease centered.
3. Learn about the patient as a person, using the FIFE mnemonic:
    a. **F**eelings: "What are you most concerned about?"
    b. **I**deas: "What do you think might be going on?"
    c. **F**unctioning: "How has your illness affected you day to day?"
    d. **E**xpectations: "What are your expectations about what might happen or can be done?"
B. Developmental tasks of the dying should be acknowledged and assisted while identifying goals of care
1. Renewed personhood (sense of meaning)
2. Closure to relationships (including forgiveness)
3. Closure to worldly affairs (work, finances)
4. Surrender to the transcendent (adapting to role as patient)
C. Meaning
1. The universal search for purpose, connection, and wholeness; four aspects can affect a patient's sense of meaning:
    a. Purpose: Can my goals be achieved or fulfilled?
    b. Value: Who will remember me?
    c. Efficacy: Sense or reality of losing control.
    d. Self-worth: I don't deserve this, am I being punished?
2. Methods that may help enhance a sense of meaning and hope:
    a. Controlling pain and symptoms
    b. Minimizing psychological distress by reinforcing purpose, value, and roles, and relaying life stories
    c. Relationship building and improving communication
        i. Patients may want to write stories, take video and pictures, or make other memorabilia for their surviving family members or friends
    d. Relaxation via poetry, art, and music
    e. Empathic presence
        i. Reinforce that the patient will not be abandoned by the healthcare team.
        ii. Allow patient and family freedom to question and get angry.
        iii. Use "I wish" statements and focus on what you can do.
        iv. Avoid statements such as, "there is nothing else I can do," or "there is no hope."

    f. Foster hope by focusing on achievable goals
      i. Use "hope" as a verb. Hope can range from hope for a cure to hope for more time to hope for symptom relief to hope for a comfortable and peaceful death.
      ii. Identify short-term and practical goals.
      iii. If unable to identify achievable short-term or practical goals, focus on goals such as achieving inner peace, making sure that family will be okay, and reassurance that unfinished business will be taken care of.
    g. Goal setting involves looking at 4 items
      i. Whose goals are they: the patient's, surrogate's, or physician's? Are they in the patient's best interest?
        (A) Best interest is typically defined by the patient.
      ii. Are the goals achievable?
      iii. Are the goals beneficial?
      iv. Are the results measurable? Identify clear, time-limited markers to see if the goal is being achieved and determine what will be done based on the results of a time-limited trial.

BAD NEWS

I. Serious findings, poor prognosis, or nearing end-of-life
  A. Bad news should be provided by the physician in charge, along with facilitators or other team members for supporting both physician and patient.
    1. It should not be provided by other nonphysician team members.
    2. Family members should not find out before the patient.
      a. Potential surgical findings should be discussed with the patient prior to the surgery or imaging study. By asking patients how they would like results or information delivered. This can resolve scenarios in which families do not wish for the patient to know the findings.
    3. Ideally, advance directives should be completed and reviewed prior to surgery.
    4. When giving bad news, remember the patient needs to feel in control. When asked, patients said they were thankful for the following:
      a. Physicians who were empathic, yet direct and clear
      b. An available clear diagnosis
      c. An explanation of the prognosis and how it relates to their quality of life
      d. The inclusion of a trusted family member or friend
      e. The offer to ask questions
      f. A disclosure that was neither overly optimistic or pessimistic
      g. A physician who was practical with a clear plan for what to do next

5. When delivering bad news, utilize mnemonic "SPIKES":
   a. **S**etting: Arrange the atmosphere (private room, shake patient's hand first, always sit down, silence electronic devices).
   b. **P**erception: Find out what the patient knows.
   c. **I**nformation desired: Find out what they want to know.
   d. **K**nowledge:
      i. Share: If appropriate utilize so-called "warning shots" ("I'm afraid the situation is more serious than we thought.").
      ii. Align: Seek understanding and expect to repeat yourself a lot, sometimes answering the same questions over multiple visits.
      iii. Educate: Ask for permission to offer a clear diagnosis and also ask for permission to provide a clear prognosis. If permission given then use language the patient and family will understand when relaying that information. Then pause and finally check for understanding. If patient is dying, then say "dying." Avoid withholding information unless a patient has stated he/she does not want to hear certain information and delegates that duty to a surrogate.
   e. **E**mpathy:
      i. Avoid saying, "there is nothing more that I can do," and discuss what can be done or the care that is available, such as symptom control.
      ii. Avoid saying, "I'm sorry there is no cure."
      iii. Use more accurate verbiage with "I wish" statements such as "I wish there was a cure," "I wish we could do that," "I wish there were better treatments for your cancer," or "I wish it were different" (since in reality you do wish those things).
   f. **S**olutions: Summarize and provide solutions. Include a clear safety net. Make a plan and provide it to patient and surrogates in writing. It should be clear on what to do or what will be done if the plan does not work, and on what signs indicate that a plan is or is not working.
B. Responding to anger.
   1. Stay calm, do not get defensive, and do not correct or clarify immediately; instead, acknowledge and understand the feeling and clarify the content.
      a. Remember, even if the problem cannot be fixed, such as an inevitable death, you should provide reassurance that your patient will not be abandoned.
      b. Fear is the most common source of anger and should be explored without withdrawing or getting angry yourself.

2. Limit self-disclosure.
   a. This is not about you or your similar life experiences; it is about your patient. Make sure to keep the conversation focused on the patient.
   b. Maintain professional boundaries and avoid complaining about colleagues, organizations, and society, as doing so will likely increase distress.
3. Utilize the mnemonic "NURSE":
   a. **N**ame the emotion, without telling them what they are feeling.
      i. "It sounds like...", "Some people have told me they feel..."
   b. **U**nderstand by demonstrating empathy.
      i. "It must be hard to..." "I cannot understand what this must be like, can you further describe..."
   c. **R**espect by demonstrating empathy.
      i. "I'm so impressed that you...", "I see that faith is a very important part of your life..."
   d. **S**upport and tell the patient/family they will be supported.
      i. "Our team will continue to..."
   e. **E**xplore and discuss available options; brainstorm ideas.
      i. "Tell me more about..."

THE FAMILY

I. **Family systems theory**
   A. The patient is the unit of treatment, and the family is the unit of understanding.
   B. The whole (patient and family) is greater than the individual units, and a change in any unit effects every other unit.
   C. Who is part of the family is defined by the patient.
II. **Enhanced autonomy**
   A. Autonomy that is supported by exploring both the patient's and family's values and goals.
   B. Involves clearly integrating these values and goals with the medical facts and offering a recommendation that might achieve or move closer to these goals.
   C. Providing a clear recommendation can help remove guilt that family members may feel (e.g., making a medical decision without a clear physician recommendation).
III. **The family meeting**
   A. Its purpose is to allow patients and family to review what has been happening.
      1. Review diagnosis, treatments, and prognosis.
      2. Clarify goals of care.
      3. Review options available.

4. Make decisions on how best to proceed.
5. Clarify clearly what information needs to be reviewed and what decisions needs to be clarified when scheduling the meeting.

B. Utilize the "SPIKES" mnemonic as with delivering bad news:

1. **S**etting: In a quiet and private room, sit down in a circle with family members, avoiding unnecessary barriers. The decisional patient can help guide whether the meeting should take place with their participation or not.

2. **P**erception: Utilize "ask-tell-ask" or "chunk and check" methods.
   a. Get started by utilizing the "AIDET" mnemonic:
      i. **A**cknowledge people: Thank everyone for their time and demonstrating how important the patient is.
      ii **I**ntroduce everyone.
      iii. **D**uration: Talk about how long the meeting will be and touch on what everyone would like to discuss.
      iv. **E**xplain (continue below with rest of SPIKES mnemonic).
      v. **T**hanks: Thank everyone and offer the opportunity for follow-up.
   b. *Ask* about what they know, *tell* by confirming or clarifying facts and perceptions, *ask* for understanding.
   c. Keep questions and statements open ended, and keep checking until their understanding or emotion has been fully expressed and understood.

3. **I**nformation desired: Clarify what patient and family would like to know more about.

4. **K**nowledge: Again, utilize "ask-tell-ask" or "chunk and check" to confirm understanding.
   a. Review advance directives if available.
   b. Review new or updated physician findings, including what is and is not working.
   c. Review prognosis (functional status, symptom burden, and anticipated survival, such as in days to weeks, weeks to months, or months to years).

5. **E**mpathy: Utilize "I wish" statements whenever appropriate.

6. **S**olutions: "Have you thought about what you would like to do if things continue to get worse?"
   a. Review available options that meet the patient's values and goals. Summarize the discussion (consensus, disagreements, decisions, next steps, follow-up meetings) and make sure a family spokesperson has been identified and documented in chart.
   b. Avoid framing choices as "doing everything" or "withdrawing" treatments. This implies that the options are doing less than "everything" and that the team or the family is "giving up"

and that by withdrawing a specific treatment we are withdrawing "care" (we always care for the patient and palliative care can be "aggressive" or "intensive"). Refocus the discussion on what is not working, what is working, what can be done for the patient, and what you recommend.

C. Other scenarios:
   1. "Dad's a fighter," or "Mom would never give up"
      a. Do not argue over facts. What is happening medically is happening, and you should not repeat these facts unless asked to. Acknowledge, understand, and respect that their loved one is a fighter and has fought hard. Use "I wish" statements, and explore the emotion behind these statements.
   2. "I want you to do everything"
      a. This should be clarified with goals of care in mind as the statement in itself is not complete ("I want you to do everything to..."). Emotions will be high and personalities amplified when family members are discussing a loved one who is dying.
   3. "We are waiting for a miracle"
      a. Understand, respect, and explore the emotions behind the statement. Allow family members to process information. It may take several meetings to process information and grieve. This allows more time to see the patient's progress, lack of progress, or continued decline. Make sure family members are supported (chaplains, social services, palliative care).
   4. Refusal to participate or talk
      a. Remember that one needs to be emotionally ready to discuss end-of-life issues. This requires time and regular opportunities for discussion that will allow patients and families time to reflect on the information and the effect it has on their lives.
   5. "Don't tell my mom"
      a. This request is often made out of love in an attempt to protect the patient from emotional harm.
      b. Current professional standards state that patients have the right to information in order to make informed decisions. However, this does not mean that patients should be forced to hear unwanted information.
      c. Clarify the request and be empathic. Normalize the concerns (worried about harming patient) and understand what they fear might happen if information is or is not shared.
      d. Tell them the benefits of sharing the information, because most patients want to know and will want to discuss it and their concerns about dying.
         i. Withholding information isolates patients and prevents them from planning and truly saying goodbye.

    e. Brainstorm solutions such as sharing limited information or asking the patient how much they would like to know or if they would prefer doctors talk with a surrogate instead.

6. Conflicts

    a. Minimize conflict by keeping discussions patient centered. Learn the patient's and family's stories, and focus on their concerns. Acknowledge and understand emotions. Refocus discussions on what was identified as being important to the patient. When conflicts remain, utilize these principled negotiation techniques:

       i. Separate the problem from personalities.

         (A) Not problems: Doctors are giving up, family is in denial, patient is being unreasonable, or spouse is acting out. These are opinions about personalities.

         (B) Problem: The patient is dying. Treatments are not working or requested treatments will not improve quality and/or quantity of life.

       ii. Clearly identify and express interests.

         (A) Family wants what is best; identify what that means. Is it about preventing starvation or gasping for air? Is it about faith? Is it about fear of death or abandonment?

         (B) The medical team wants to provide the best and most beneficial medical care, while avoiding harm and undesired treatments.

    b. Brainstorm solutions, such as time-limited trials or other ways of meeting mutually identified interests. Focus on shared goals, not on what will not or cannot be done. We all have our own values and cultures, and our own view of what constitutes a good death, and respecting these differences is important.

    c. Obtain formal ethics consultation if conflict remains or is anticipated.

D. Summary:

    1. Get to know the patient better and how they have been doing recently.

    2. Determine what the patient and family know and want to know.

    3. Confirm you are understanding what they understand.

    4. Review the medical status and prognosis.

    5. Make decisions with the patient or surrogate, but allow the family to ask questions and discuss alone if desired.

    6. Make sure the physician has provided a clear recommendation if desired and that the patient and family know they will not be abandoned if they do not follow the recommendation.

    7. Encourage everyone to hope for the best while preparing for the worst.

3 ■ ETHICAL DECISION MAKING

ETHICAL PRINCIPLES

I. Clinical ethics
   A. Palliative medicine specialists and clinical ethicists/ethics committee consultants share overlapping expertise.
      1. Both have expertise in conducting family meetings, having difficult conversations, shared decision making, advance care planning, and end-of-life decision making.
      2. Palliative medicine physicians have the medical and clinical training, background, and expertise to assist patients and families in navigating very complicated medical situations.
   B. All teams, including palliative care teams, are expected to honor and respect a patient's informed treatment decisions.
      1. Teams should be value neutral and focus on providing relevant information and supporting the patient in his/her ongoing decision-making needs.
      2. Palliative medicine recommendations are made to prevent and relieve suffering and support the best possible quality of life, not to hasten or postpone death.
      3. Do not expect patients to alter their fundamental life philosophies based on the team's opinion of what is good for them.
         a. A patient's emotional suffering may be greater than their physical suffering, which plays a role in decision making.
         b. By allowing patients permission to be true to themselves, you are still participating in their existential healing.
   C. A principle-based approach is a predominant theory in clinical ethics: These principles should be considered and balanced with the overall goals of medicine (to cure, to care, to comfort).
      1. Autonomy: Informed consent or informed refusal.
      2. Beneficence: Will the proposed intervention benefit the patient?
      3. Nonmaleficence: Will the proposed intervention needlessly create a harm?
         a. This is different from negligence, which states that there is a duty to the patient, that duty was breached, and a harm was caused by the breach.
      4. Justice: Concerns issues of fairness, such as allocation of scarce resources

ETHICS CONSULTATION

I. **Goals**
   A. Assure equitable attention to patient's rights, shared decision making, fair policies, and physician integrity, and enhance the ethical tenor of the institution.

II. **Guidelines**
   A. Everyone with moral concern or important voices in the situation should be present and closely involved, or have their values understood during the consultative process.
   B. Physician responsibilities
   1. When value conflicts arise, remember that clinical guidelines are not necessarily applicable to this particular patient. Document why or why not.
   2. The physician should evaluate the situation and make a clear recommendation appropriate for the patient.
   3. Knowing when average statistics that form the basis of guidelines are applicable or not is part of the art of medicine.
   4. When the physician makes a clear recommendation, the patient is the best person to assess the risks, benefits, goals, and costs of treatment (in the face of inevitable clinical uncertainty).
      a. Physician recommendations ideally are made based on the medical facts and the patient's values, however they can be biased by the physician's personal values.
      b. Having an independent evaluation by an ethics team that is not part of the treating medical team helps minimize the possible intrusion of personal or group bias.

III. **Approaches and models**
   A. Approach
   1. A number of different approaches exist. With an authoritarian approach, the ethicist functions as the primary moral decision maker, usurping the shared decision-making process and the authority usually afforded to patient, family members, and healthcare professionals. With a pure consensus approach, the ethicist attempts to obtain agreement from all parties involved with a patient. While building agreement is appealing, this approach may not account for significant ethical values and legal norms if they are not represented among those participating in the process.
   2. The American Society for Bioethics and Humanities (ASBH) recommends the ethics facilitation approach. The consultant's goal is to "elucidate issues, aid effective communication, and integrate the perspectives of the relevant stakeholders." It helps clarify uncertain values and facilitates a resolution between all parties. The ASBH core competencies acknowledge that "there is a fine line between educating (which may involve some degree of persuasion) and manipulating." Having a clear

mediation/facilitation process helps reduce the risk that the consultant will unduly influence or manipulate the outcome by ensuring that all voices are empowered. The following is expected from an ethics consultant:

a. Clarify the ethical questions.
b. Gather information.
c. Clarify concepts.
d. Clarify normative issues (societal values, law, ethical standards, and institutional policies).
e. Identify the ethical issue (may be different from the initial question).
f. Identify a range of ethically acceptable options (avoid providing a single option when multiple options exist, or if providing only a single recommendation, explain why other options are not ethically valid).
g. Facilitate ethical resolution between all parties by identifying decision makers, clarifying all parties' own values, and facilitating understanding of the medical facts between the physicians and patients/surrogates.
   i. For example, the consultant can ask physicians to reframe information in a manner that might be easier to understand.

B. Models
   1. Single ethicist: When questions must be answered urgently
      a. Should have advanced training in healthcare ethics consultation.
   2. Consultation teams: When several moral voices would be helpful
      a. All members should be trained in basic clinical bioethics, with a least one member having advanced training.
   3. Full committee: For particularly controversial consultations in which many moral voices would be helpful
      a. A subcommittee of the full committee would likely be available at any one time.
      b. All members should have some basic training in clinical bioethics with at least one member with advanced training.

IV. **Protocol for ethics consultation**
   A. After request is made
      1. If a request is made for an ethics consultation, the assumption is that an ethical conflict exists.
      2. Several broad categories of ethical questions exist:
         a. Shared decision making
         b. End-of-life practices
         c. Beginning-of-life practices
         d. Privacy and confidentiality
         e. Professionalism
         f. Fair resource allocation (institutional- or societal-level determinations)

g. Business and management practices
h. Everyday workplace practices
i. Research practices
3. The ethicist will assess if the concern is ethical in nature or best handled by another party.

B. Practical steps for performing an ethics consultation
1. Gather relevant information.
a. What are the facts of the case? One method to frame the information gathered is to utilize Jonsen and Siegler's 4-box method:
i. Medical indications: Diagnosis, prognosis, acute/chronic, treatment goals, probabilities of success, plans if treatment fails (principles of beneficence and nonmaleficence)
ii. Patient preferences: Intact decisional capacity, treatment preferences, informed consent/refusal, use of appropriate standards by surrogate, respect of patient's right to choose (principle of autonomy)
iii. Quality of life: Prospects of returning to a normal life with or without treatment, deficits if treatment succeeds, identification of provider biases, might quality of life be considered undesirable? Are there plans to forego current treatments or to pursue comfort care? (principles of beneficence, nonmaleficence, and autonomy)
iv. Contextual features: Family issues and biases; financial, religious, or cultural factors; resource allocation considerations; provider or institutional conflicts of interest (principles of justice, loyalty, and fairness)
2. How should the issues be framed? What is the ethical question?
a. Consider basic ethical principles and the goals of medicine in light of the values and preferences identified.
3. Consider options.
a. Were any precedents or prior broad moral consensus identified?
b. What could be done, and what should be done?
c. Care is not optional; it is always provided no matter the patient's goals or the achievable goals of medicine; what changes is the type of care. In other words we never remove, withdraw, or stop care.
d. Are there ethical arguments against what should be done?
4. Make a clear recommendation that treats all parties in an ethical manner.
a. Focus on fair processes and relationships rather than on outcomes.
b. Document in the medical record who requested consultation and why, who participated in the consultation, the findings, clarified values, and final recommendation(s).
5. Check and follow-up to determine if the course selected is working; readdress as needed.

SHARED DECISION MAKING

I. **Decisional capacity assessment**
   A. Decision making should occur with patients and/or surrogates that have intact decision-making capacity.
   B. The level of capacity needed depends on the importance of the question at hand.
      1. Selecting which arm to use for blood draws would require minimal capacity, whereas consenting to or refusing an amputation would require maximal capacity.
      2. Capacity may fluctuate during times of the day or on different days, such as with patients in delirium.
   C. Intact capacity can legally be determined by any physician.
      1. If unclear or possibly affected by psychiatric illness, then ask for a formal psychiatric evaluation.
      2. Findings of the capacity evaluation should be documented by the physician and should be noted if situational or limited to a certain decision.
      3. Capacity assessment is not a competence determination, which is a legal determination determined by a judge.
   D. Criteria: Patient or surrogate should be able to understand, deliberate, and communicate a decision.
      1. Understand: Appreciating and comprehending the situation including its importance and seriousness of the facts; they can be tested by the ability to paraphrase (not recite) back the pertinent medical facts.
      2. Deliberate: The patient is able to weigh the pros and cons of the decision in a defensible manner, in the context of his/her values.
      3. Communicate: The patient can express a decision clearly and consistently over time.

II. **Legal concerns**
   A. Advance care planning documentation: A patient may have completed some level of advance care planning and recorded the planning in a legal document.
      • Documents vary by state and may include documentation of surrogates, healthcare treatment, and physician orders that operationalize advance directives.
         a. Advance directive documents that include treatment preferences should be reviewed and confirmed if they still reflect patient's current wishes.
         b. Physician order documents: Physician/medical orders for life-sustaining treatment or scope of treatment (POLST/MOLST/POST/MOST) are legal orders that can be acted upon by any healthcare provider and as such, should be reviewed and signed by a physician and the patient/surrogate following discussion and review. The form is portable across healthcare settings including home and may be revoked and revised by the patient/surrogate working with a physician at any time.

B. Legally identified surrogates:
1. Surrogate decision makers have the same authority and responsibility for decision making as the incapacitated patient the surrogate represents.
2. Institutional policies usually define the process for identifying an appropriate surrogate for incapacitated patients without one.
3. An identified surrogate should have decision-making capacity, be readily available for decision making, and utilize either of these 2 criteria in promoting the patient's preferences and welfare:
   a. Substituted judgment: Based on previously expressed statements or actions of the patient
   b. The "best interests" standard: What a reasonable person in similar circumstances would decide

III. Informed consent

A. Demonstrates respect for patient autonomy and allows for a patient to deliberate information and provide voluntary consent.
B. It is not documenting and signing a form, but a discussion between patient and physician tailored to that particular decision.
C. Discussions and documentation should be free of coercion and include the following items:
1. Current diagnosis and natural course without any interventions
2. Options that meet the patient's goals of care and/or improve prognosis
   a. Include a discussion of the risks, benefits, complications, and anticipated effects on patient's life
3. Alternatives including option to allow a natural course without further interventions
4. Physician recommendation based on clinical judgment and knowledge of patient's goals and values

WITHHOLDING VERSUS WITHDRAWING TREATMENT

I. No ethical difference

A. Psychologically or emotionally, however, it may be easier to withhold than to withdraw treatment.
B. Withholding treatment often requires clearer clinical evidence, discussions, and decision making due to natural clinical uncertainty or uncertainty as to patient's values.
C. Withdrawing treatment requires clinical evidence that treatment is failing or not meeting the patient's goals of care.
D. When reasonable uncertainty exists, a time-limited trial with specific outcome measures should be considered.
   - A trial of artificial nutrition with objective outcomes such as improved pressure ulcer healing, albumin, weight, or functional status, and avoiding harm such as persistent diarrhea, worsening heart failure, or increasing aspirations, secretions, or edema

II. **Care is always provided**
   A. One should not discuss withholding or withdrawing care as this is not true.
   B. Always identify the medical intervention(s) being discussed when talking about withholding or withdrawing a specific medical intervention.

DEATH

I. **Death**
   A. Death is defined as an irreversible cessation of the circulatory and respiratory systems or of functions of the entire brain, including the brain stem
      1. No published reports of neurological recovery after a person has been declared dead by the American Academy of Neurology's brain death criteria
      2. Reports of complex, spontaneous motor movements and false-positive triggering of the ventilator in patients who are still confirmed to be brain dead
   B. Brain death diagnosis (3 clinical findings)
      1. Comatose (with a known cause)
         a. Minimal acceptable observation period (undefined)
         b. Normothermic
         c. No response to noxious stimuli
      2. Absence of brain stem reflexes
         a. No pupillary, corneal, or oculocephalic/oculovestibular reflexes.
            i. Pupils typically are fixed and dilated (4–9 mm).
            ii. Eyes should not move with head movement (ensure stable spine) or with 50 mL of ice water into external auditory canals.
         b. No grimacing or facial muscle movement in response to noxious stimulus.
         c. No pharyngeal or tracheal reflexes such as with tongue blade or tracheal suctioning.
      3. Apnea test
         a. Patient should have normal blood pressure and temperature, be euvolemic, and have normal CO_2 and oxygenation at the start. Adjust vasopressors to keep SBP ≥100 mm Hg and preoxygenate with 100% O_2 to get PaO_2 to >200 mm Hg.
         b. Reduce ventilator rate to 10 and PEEP to 5, if O_2 saturation remains >95%, then obtain baseline ABG and disconnect patient from ventilator.
         c. Deliver 100% O_2 at 6l pm via catheter placed via ET tube to level of carina.

  d. Observe for spontaneous respirations over 8–10 minutes. Stop anytime SBP <90 mm Hg or O_2 sat <85% for >30 seconds and can retry with T-piece, CPAP 10 cm H_2O, and 100% O_2 at 12l pm.

  e. If no respirations noted by abdominal or chest excursions, obtain repeat ABG at 8 minutes and if PCO_2 increased by 20 mm Hg or ≥60 mm Hg, then test is positive for brain death (and this is the time of death).

 4. Confirmatory tests

  a. Not required for diagnosis and typically do not require consent (i.e., for confirming brain death).

  b. Cerebral angiography, electroencephalography, transcranial Doppler ultrasonography, or cerebral scintigraphy (radioisotope-based) can be considered if unclear findings based on clinical criteria or if the apnea test cannot be performed.

  c. If these tests show findings consistent with brain death, then this will be the time of death.

PHYSICIAN-ASSISTED SUICIDE AND EUTHANASIA

I. **Physician-assisted suicide**

 A. Physician provides a prescription for the lethal drug(s) with instructions for its use, but the patient is the agent who decides when and if to take it and self-administers.

II. **Euthanasia**

 A. Physician intentionally administers a lethal drug combination for the purpose of causing immediate death in a patient with a terminal, incurable, or painful disease.

III. **Legality**

 A. Most medical and nursing national and state associations prohibit physician-assisted suicide and euthanasia (even if euthanasia were legal).

 B. U.S. state laws differ with regard to physician-assisted suicide, but euthanasia (both voluntary and involuntary) is illegal in all states.

4 ■ PROGNOSTICATION

I. Background

A. Physicians universally overestimate prognosis and the longer the doctor/patient relationship, the more inaccurate the prognostication.

B. Metastatic cancer is most predictable, however conditions like heart failure and chronic obstructive pulmonary disease are very difficult to prognosticate, and this should be part of the discussion.

C. Consider asking for a second opinion from a physician not related to the patient who can provide an unbiased opinion based on the clinical information alone.

D. Prognostication helps identify which patients would most benefit from additional supportive services and advance care planning.

E. Providing details on scales used often is not helpful to patients, but rather use them to guide providers in understanding and delivering the big picture.

II. Common scales in use to assist in prognostication

A. Karnofsky performance scale (KPS): If <40, median survival is 3 months.

B. Palliative performance scale (PPS): Based on the KPS: For patients requiring admission to hospital-based palliative care units, if PPS ≤60, median survival can be measured in weeks.

C. Eastern Cooperative Oncology Group (ECOG), or WHO/Zubrod score: If >3, median survival is 3 months.

D. Palliative prognostic score (PaP): For estimating prognosis suspected to be measured in weeks; validated for terminally ill solid-tumor cancer patients; also found to be reliable for those with organ failure, AIDS, and neurological diseases.

E. Palliative prognostic index (PPI): For estimating prognosis suspected to be measured in weeks; validated for terminally ill cancer patients.

F. An online tool for elderly patients is available at www.eprognosis.org.

HOSPICE CRITERIA

I. Prognostication guidelines

A. Surprise question: Would I be surprised if this patient died in the next year? If the answer is no, then consider identifying when and if hospice services may benefit the patient and ensuring concurrent palliative services are provided.

B. Prognostication tools are continuing to improve and communication should occur with the patient's primary treating physicians for updated prognostic information.

C. Use current available information to provide an estimated prognosis.

D. Some of these guidelines (such as dementia) have not been found to be highly predictive, but Medicare may deny claims if deviations from traditional criteria are not adequately explained.

TABLE 4.1 Hospice Criteria

Disease	Primary Criteria (required)	Secondary Criteria (helpful)
General Guidelines (terminal illness not due to a specific single illness)	Rapid decline over 3–6 months (document signs, symptoms) PPS ≤50% (mainly sit/lie, not working, needing moderate assistance)	Involuntary weight loss >10%/6 months or albumin ≤2.5 g/dL
Adult Failure to Thrive	PPS ≤40% (mainly bedbound) BMI <22 kg/m² Not responding to adequate nutritional supplementation (or refuses nutritional support)	Malnutrition (albumin ≤2.5, total cholesterol <160, anemia, leukopenia) Apathy Anorexia "Multifactorial decline"
Cancer	Extensive disease PPS ≤70% (reduced ambulation, unable to work outside home) Declining despite life-prolonging therapy OR refuses further life-prolonging therapy	Hypercalcemia >12 mg/dL Weight loss >5%/3 months Cachexia Recurrence of disease after initial definitive treatment Symptoms of advanced disease (such as nausea, anemia, ascites, pleural effusion)
Dementia	FAST (Functional Assessment Stage) 7C or worse (cannot walk without assistance, speaking ≤6 words, incontinent (bowel/bladder), assistance with activities of daily living AND Within 6 months infection (aspiration pneumonia, pyelonephritis, or septicemia), fevers, stage 3 or 4 pressure ulcers, OR malnutrition despite adequate supplementation (weight loss >10% or albumin <2.5 g/dL)	n/a

(continues)

TABLE 4.1 (*continued*)

Disease	Primary Criteria (required)	Secondary Criteria (helpful)
Heart Disease	Heart failure (NYHA Class IV) On optimal heart failure treatment OR has resting angina (nitrate resistant and not invasive candidate or refuses invasive procedures)	EF ≤20% Dysrhythmias despite optimal treatment Refractory syncope (due to cardiac etiology) Stroke due to cardiac etiology (embolic) History of cardiac resuscitation (CPR) Concurrent HIV
HIV/AIDS	CD4+ <25 cell/mcl OR viral load >100,000/ml AIDS diagnosis (CNS lymphoma, refractory wasting [>33% loss of lean body mass], MAC infection, progressive multifocal leukoencephalopathy, systemic lymphoma, visceral KS, renal failure [not dialysis candidate], cryptosporidium infection, OR refractory toxoplasmosis) PPS ≤50% (mainly sit/lie, not working, needing moderate assistance)	Foregoing HAART or prophylaxis Diarrhea >1 year NYHA Class IV heart failure Albumin ≤2.5 g/dL Age >50 years Ongoing substance abuse
Liver Diseases	INR >1.5 Albumin <2.5 g/dL Cirrhosis symptoms (refractory ascites, history of spontaneous bacterial peritonitis, hepatorenal syndrome, refractory hepatic encephalopathy, or history of recurrent variceal bleeding) Declines or not a liver transplant candidate (if a transplant candidate can meet criteria and utilize hospice services until liver found, if ever)	Malnutrition Muscle wasting Active alcoholism (>80 g ethanol/day) Hepatocellular carcinoma HBsAg positive Refractory hepatitis C
Pulmonary Diseases	Severe chronic lung disease (dyspnea at rest, refractory to bronchodilators, bed/chair bound, fatigue, chronic cough) Progression of disease (increasing office, home, ED, or hospital visits) Within 3 months (especially if on supplemental O_2) pO_2 <55 or O_2 sat <88% OR pCO_2 >50	Cor pulmonale with right heart failure Unintentional progressive weight loss FEV1 <30% of predicted Resting tachycardia (>100)

(continued)

TABLE 4.1 (*continued*)

Disease	Primary Criteria (required)	Secondary Criteria (helpful)
Neurological Diseases	Chronic degenerating neurological condition (ALS, MS, myasthenia gravis, muscular dystrophies, Parkinson's disease) Respiratory failure (dyspnea at rest, VC <30% of predicted [note for ALS patients: PEG maybe helpful if VC >50%, bipap or tracheostomy maybe helpful if VC <30%], O_2 at rest, AND declines invasive mechanical ventilation) OR Rapid disease progression (functional decline) with either 12 months of progressive malnutrition or life-threatening infection/complication (aspiration pneumonia, pyelonephritis, sepsis, fevers, stage 3 or 4 pressure ulcer)	—
Renal Failure	Not a renal replacement therapy candidate (or declines) Creatinine clearance <10 mL/min (<15 for diabetics) Serum creatinine >8 mg/dL (>6 for diabetics)	Chronic renal failure: uremia, oliguria (UO <400 mL/24 h), refractory hyperkalemia (>7 mEq/L), uremic pericarditis, hepatorenal syndrome, refractory fluid overload) Acute renal failure: respiratory failure (requiring mechanical ventilation), nonrenal cancer, advanced chronic lung, cardiac, or liver disease
Stroke or Coma	PPS ≤40% (mainly bedbound) Malnutrition (≥10% weight loss/6 months or ≥7.5% in 3 months, albumin <2.5 g/dL, or inability to decrease respiratory aspiration events)	Acute: On 3rd day of coma (from any etiology) 3 of the following 4 criteria: Abnormal brain stem Nonverbal No withdrawal to pain Serum creatinine >1.5 g/dL Chronic: Within 1 year: aspiration pneumonia, pyelonephritis, sepsis, fevers, stage 3 or 4 pressure ulcers

INTENSIVE CARE UNIT

I. **Cardiac arrest resulting in CPR**
   A. Patients already in ICU at time of arrest
      1. On vasopressors at the time: 9.3% survival to discharge (3.9% to home)
      2. Not on vasopressors at the time: 21.2% (8.5% to home)
      3. Overall: 15.9% survival to hospital discharge
II. **Prognosis for prolonged ventilation (ProVent score): Measure at 21 days (or ≥3 weeks)**

TABLE 4.2 Prognosis for Prolonged Ventilation (ProVent) Score of Both Sexes from All Ethnicities, Listed from Most to Least

Criteria (at 3 weeks)	Score
Age ≥50 years old?	1
Currently on vasopressors?	1
Current platelet count ≤150,000 K	1
Currently on hemodialysis	1
1-year mortality (%)	Total Score
15	0
42	1
88	2
95	3
100	4

Source: Adapted from Carson, S. S., Garrett, J., Hanson, L. C., et al. (2008). A prognostic model for one-year mortality in patients requiring prolonged mechanical ventilation. *Critical Care Medicine*, 36(7), 2061–2069.

DISEASE BASED GUIDELINES

I. **Cancer**
   A. Performance status is most predictive.
      1. If spending >50% of the time sitting or lying down, then 3-month median survival.
      2. Dyspnea due to the cancer is second most predictive.
   B. <6 months if metastatic solid cancer, acute leukemia, or high-grade lymphoma and no plans for systemic chemotherapy (except for metastatic breast and prostate cancer if performance status is good).
   C. <6 months prognosis if has malignant ascites, pleural effusion, or malignant bowel obstruction.
   D. 3–6 months if multiple brain metastases with radiation.
      1. 1–2 months without.
   E. <3 months if carcinomatous meningitis.
   F. <2 months if malignant pericardial effusion or malignant hypercalcemia (except for newly diagnosed breast cancer or myeloma).

TABLE 4.3 Top 10 Deadliest Cancers of Both Sexes from All Ethnicities, Listed from Most to Least

Lung
Prostate
Breast (Female)
Colon and Rectum
Pancreas
Ovary
Leukemias
Non-Hodgkin's Lymphoma
Liver and Intrahepatic Bile Duct
Urinary Bladder

Source: Data from SEER Cancer Statistics Review, 1975–2009 and United States Cancer Statistics: 1999–2008 Incidence and Mortality.

II. Chronic obstructive lung disease
- ADO index (Age–Dyspnea–Obstruction): 3-year prognostication tool for poor functional status patients.

TABLE 4.4 ADO Index

Criteria	Score
Age	
50–59	1
60–69	2
70–79	3
80–89	4
≥90	5
Dyspnea (Medical Research Council Scale)	
MRC 2 (dyspnea with <4 metabolic equivalents but at usual pace, recovering quickly upon stopping)	1
MRC 3 (dyspnea at slow walk, taking few minutes to recover)	2
MRC 4 (dyspnea with light activity like dressing or leaving house)	3
Obstruction (FEV1 %)	
36–64%	1
≤35%	2

(continues)

TABLE 4.4 (*continued*)

Criteria	Score
Longstanding severe COPD	First admission with moderate to severe COPD

Points	3-year mortality risk (%)	Points	3-year mortality risk
0	7.2 (2.7–17.9)	0	3 (0.9–9)
1	9.9 (4.4–20.6)	1	4 (1.6–10)
2	13.5 (7.2–23.8)	2	5.4 (2.7–10.9)
3	18.1 (11.4–27.5)	3	7.3 (4.3–12.1)
4	23.9 (17.4–31.8)	4	9.8 (6.8–13.9)
5	30.8 (24.8–37.4)	5	12.9 (9.6–17.1)
6	38.7 (32–45.7)	6	16.9 (12–23.3)
7	47.2 (37.9–56.6)	7	21.8 (13.7–32.8)
8	55.9 (43.1–68)	8	27.6 (15.2–44.9)
9	64.2 (47.8–77.8)	9	34.3 (16.7–57.9)
10	71.8 (52.4–85.4)	10	41.7 (18–70)

Source: Adapted from Puhan, M. A., Garcia-Aymerich, J., Frey, M., et al. (2009). Expansion of the prognostic assessment of patients with chronic obstructive pulmonary disease: the updated BODE index and the ADO index. *The Lancet,* 374(9691), 704–711.

III. **Heart failure**
  A. Very difficult to prognosticate due to an unpredictable trajectory combined with a high incidence of sudden death.
  B. A web-based calculator is available at www.seattleheartfailuremodel. org for chronic heart failure.
  C. A web-based calculator for 7-day mortality for acute heart failure is available at www.acponline.org/journals/annals/extras/ehmrg/.

IV. **End-stage liver disease**
  A. Child-Pugh class: Can be used to assist in assessing prognosis of chronic liver disease and perioperative mortality.
  B. Model for end-stage liver disease (MELD) score can be calculated and may be more or less predictive than the Child-Pugh score.
    1. Does not require clinical assessment of ascites and encephalopathy, and is calculated based on 3 easily measurable variables: INR, bilirubin, and creatinine (which is assumed to be 4 if on hemodialysis).
    2. Web-based calculator can be found at www.mayoclinic.org/ meld/mayomodel6.html.
  C. Severe hepatorenal syndrome: If moderate to severe then prognosis is measured in weeks (8–10 weeks with therapy); if mild (creatinine stabilizes around 1.5–2 mg/dL) then prognosis is measured in months (around 6 months).

TABLE 4.5 Child-Pugh Class

Criteria	Score
Total bilirubin (mg/dL)	
<2	1
2–3	2
>3	3
Total bilirubin for primary sclerosing cholangitis or primary biliary cirrhosis	
≤4	1
≤10	2
>10	3
Serum albumin (g/dL)	
>3.5	1
2.8–3.5	2
<2.8	3
INR	
<1.7	1
1.71–2.20	2
>2.20	3
Ascites	
None	1
Controlled with medications	2
Refractory to medications	3
Hepatic encephalopathy	
None	1
Grade I–II or controlled with medications	2
Grade III–IV or refractory	3

Class	Life expectancy	Peri-Opmortality	Total points
A	15–20 months	10%	5–6
B	4–14 months	30%	7–9
C	1–3 months	82%	10–15

Source: Adapted from Durand, F. & Valla, D. (2005). Assessment of the prognosis of cirrhosis: Child-Pugh versus MELD. *Journal of Hepatology,* 42(Suppl 1), S100–S107.

V. **End-stage renal disease**
   A. Overall 1-year mortality for patients on hemodialysis is 25%.
      - Charlson comorbidity index may be utilized to estimate 1-year mortality.
   B. Online calculator that can estimate 6- and 12-month mortality is available at http://touchcalc.com/calculators/sq.

VI. **Dementia**
   A. See hospice criteria (see Table 4.1).
   B. The classification of terminal dementia should be reserved for patients who have lost the ability to communicate, ambulate, swallow, and maintain continence.

VII. **For nursing home patients**
   A. The Porock 6-month risk can be calculated and is available online at http://www.eprognosis.org.

5 ■ CULTURAL AND RELIGIOUS CONCERNS

ETHNIC VIEWS

TABLE 5.1 Ethnic Views of Suffering and Dying

Cultural Identity	View of Pain or Suffering	Terminal Illness and Death
Native American	Maybe kept private, may not report pain but rather feeling "uncomfortable."	Some cultures prefer to not openly discuss terminal status as negative thoughts may hasten loss. May prefer hospital based death due to minimizing contact with the dying.
Arab or Middle Eastern	Expressive about pain and suffering. Explore meaning.	Family members may protect patient from terminal diagnosis. Hospital-based death often preferred.
Black/African	May fear pain medications due to fear of addiction. Suffering may be God's punishment or will, or work of the devil. May respond to a FACES pain scale better than a numerical scale.	Sometimes terminal status shared with patient by oldest relative. Some may believe that death in the home brings bad luck.
Chinese	May not complain of pain, may prefer acupressure or acupuncture. May respond to a FACES pain scale better than a numerical pain scale.	Families prefer that key medical information and decisions be shared with the identified head of the household (ordinarily the most senior male member). Patient and family may not want to talk about end-of-life directly. Doing so may be seen as wanting to hasten death. Some believe dying at home brings bad luck.
European	Strong individualistic orientation. May feel responsible for their condition and feel a need to suffer.	Varied. Common belief in heaven and hell. Growing atheistic perspective.

(continues)

TABLE 5.1 (*continued*)

Cultural Identity	View of Pain or Suffering	Terminal Illness and Death
Filipino	May not complain of pain. May fear addiction.	Families may wish to disclose terminal prognosis to the patient with a healthcare team member present. Catholics may request to receive Sacrament of the Sick. If chronic decline is anticipated may prefer home death.
Japanese	May not complain of pain. May refuse rectal route treatments. Older generation may fear addiction.	Family and patient may avoid discussing terminal prognosis, however decisions may be made by entire family. If chronic decline is anticipated may prefer home death.
Mexican	Common belief that worry hastens clinical deterioration. May not complain of pain.	Family may want to protect patient from terminal illness prognosis. May prefer home death to allow for extended family visitation and protect the patient's spirit from getting lost in the hospital.
Russian	May not ask for pain medications. May associate morphine with developing pneumonia and fear of addiction.	Family members prefer to be notified first about terminal prognosis, trying to protect patient from worrying. Home generally preferred for death.
South Asians	Muslim patients may refuse opioids unless pain severe. Hindu and Sikh patients usually will accept opioids. May respond to a FACES pain scale better than a numerical pain scale.	Family members prefer to be notified first about terminal prognosis. Many believe soul lives on and as a result may not wish to inform patient of impending death. Home preferred location of death for most.
Vietnamese	May not request pain medications.	Family members prefer to be notified first about terminal prognosis to protect patient from worrying. If chronic decline many prefer home death.

Source: Data from multiple sources including Lipson, J. G., Dibble, S. L., & Minarik, P. A. (Eds.). (2003). *Culture & Nursing Care: A Pocket Guide.* San Francisco, CA: UCSF Nursing Press.

SPIRITUAL VIEWS

TABLE 5.2 Religious Views of Suffering and Dying

Religion	View of Suffering	Death and Afterlife	Comments
Anglican/ Episcopalian (Church of England)	Suffering is the result of evil (which comes from Satan) and God allowing freedom of choice.	May request to receive Sacrament of the Sick. Varied views of heaven and hell, most believe in eternity spent in heaven or hell.	Similar to traditional Protestant belief. The doctrinal differences and ritual practices are becoming less distinct.
Buddhist	Life is a state of suffering or dissatisfaction due to desires, therefore state of mind should be selfless, free of anger, hate, or fear by ceasing to crave. Follows basic Hindu principles of reincarnation and karma. Imperative that the dying individual remain fully aware as long as possible because thoughts while passing into death influence the after death experience.	Continual rebirth until Nirvana reached (extinction of all craving). A literal afterworld in Western China.	A patient may request that non-medication pain management techniques such as meditation be maximized.
Catholic	May view suffering in a positive light (as participating in the redemptive power of Christ's suffering).	Priest should be offered. Divine judgement follows death. Those who have rejected God are condemned to be eternally separated from God (hell). Purgatory is a state of purification after death for persons ultimately destined for eternal life with God (heaven). Only those completely free from sin at the time of death are immediately with God in heaven.	—

(continues)

TABLE 5.2 (*continued*)

Religion	View of Suffering	Death and Afterlife	Comments
Christian Science	Opposed to using psychotherapy and medications, including for pain relief (healing is the will of God and not governed by the human mind or body). Sickness is the result of fear, ignorance, or sin.	Typically will refuse life support interventions. Death is adjusting to a new consciousness. Heaven and hell are states of mind with heaven representing harmony.	–
Hindu	Life in this world means suffering. Karma is a type of natural law. If one dies before reaping the effects of one's action, then reincarnation will occur.	Reincarnation (endless round of birth, death, rebirth) until the final goal of salvation is reached (joining with Brahman).	–
Islam	Total submission of the self to the will of Allah, any treatments that may hasten death are forbidden.	Death is the end of physical life and the individual exists in a type of "soul sleep" until resurrection by Allah. Many believe that only Allah can decide when someone will die, hence may request unrestricted medical support. Ideally home is preferred location of death.	–
Jehovah's Witness	Suffering may be self-inflicted or caused by Satan. A patient may request their Jehovah's Witness Hospital Liaison Committee be contacted.	Hell is the common grave of mankind, but does not exist in the literal sense. People simply cease to exist at death (annihilated). At the resurrection, those who are saved will then be brought to life.	–

(*continues*)

TABLE 5.2 (continued)

Religion	View of Suffering	Death and Afterlife	Comments
Judaism	Typically will accept medical interventions recommended to decrease suffering. Life-prolonging interventions take priority for most.	Multiple views of the afterlife exist. Death may not be end of existence. Wide variation of views on the afterlife. Religious patients may request their rabbi to assist with difficult medical decisions as various Jewish groups differ on medical interventions at the end of life.	—
Mormon	Moral evil predated Satan, and is a necessary state that allows free choice. Death/disease is a result of natural evil that occurred after the fall of Adam and Eve.	Three heavens exist where most souls will go to. A fourth location called "Outer Darkness" is similar to the traditional Christian concept of hell.	—
Protestant	Suffering is the result of evil (which originated with Satan) and God allowing freedom of choice (free will).	Traditional Protestant Christian view of heaven (eternal reward or eternal life) and hell (eternal torment or a minority believe in annihilation or eternal death). Some believe afterlife begins at moment of death, others in a type of soul sleep with afterlife beginning at the resurrection and second coming of Christ.	—
Sikh	Suffering is part of karma and should be accepted.	Life is sacred, the soul is eternal and will rejoin God at death. Most will not accept long-term life support if permanently unconscious.	—

Source: Data from Doka, K. J. (2011). Religion and spirituality: assessment and intervention. Journal of Social Work in End-of-Life & Palliative Care 7, 99–109.

I. **Some of these generalities may lead to perceived difficulty in conversations and decision making.**
- Utilize the advanced communication skills discussed in Chapter 2 to gain a deeper understanding of your patient and maximize shared decision making.

II. **Spiritual history and interventions**
   A. Spirituality describes how one ascribes meaning to life.
   - It is very personal and is the act of looking for meaning in a way that is authentically ours.
   B. Religion is based on shared beliefs and behaviors and means, "that which binds together."
   C. Religion and spirituality can both help and hurt a patient and can affect a patient's response to illness and medical interventions.
      1. Identifying, acknowledging, and treating any spiritual struggles your patient is dealing with can help them tremendously.
      2. A near universal need is to have lived a life of meaning so providing some type of existential life review can be helpful.
   D. Interventions.
      1. Spiritual screen: Typically performed by an admission clerk
         - Identifies a patient's faith affiliation and whether there are any special needs such as diet or blood product restrictions.
      2. Spiritual history: Typically done by a chaplain, nurse, social worker, or physician with the information placed in the medical record.
         a. Focuses less on what the person believes and more on how it can help them cope
         b. Information is then used to make an appropriate referral as needed.
      3. Spiritual assessment: Employed by chaplains or pastors.
         a. In-depth tools, typically more suited for an outpatient setting (nursing home, hospice, clinic) in which repeated counseling sessions may occur.
      4. Regardless of the tools used, one should show respect for the patient's expression of faith or beliefs and remember to explore the emotions behind statements of faith.

TABLE 5.3 FACT Spiritual History Assessment

F Faith	What things do you believe that give your life meaning and purpose? Do you consider yourself a spiritual person? What is your faith?
A Active Available Accessible	Are you currently active in your faith community? Is support from your faith community available to you? Have you accessed help from your faith community?
C Coping Comfort	How are you coping with your medical situation? Is your faith helping you cope? How is your faith providing comfort to you?
T Treatment plan	If coping well, then provide ongoing team support and reassess as needed.

If coping poorly, then provide one of the following treatments.

1. Direct support. If your relationship is such (you may have a prior non medical relationship with patient or a strong, long-established relationship with the patient, or you are a chaplain) and you share the same faith and if patient is welcoming to such support, then feel free to provide the support immediately (if you are comfortable doing so without imposing your personal beliefs). Interventions may range from supporting and encouraging the patient in their own faith journey to providing a prayer.

   a. Prayer

   Prayer maybe a calming influence to patients. Often fears for themselves, their family, 'why me?', 'am I being punished?' can be helped by having a sense of peace that patient's may achieve by prayer. Always ask permission, such as "would it be helpful to you if I prayed with you?" If you note any hesitation then don't pray. If they welcome it (and several studies show beneficial effects when focused on patient's needs and concerns) then pray specifically about the items the patient talked about or is worried about.

2. Faith community referral. Encourage self-referral or obtain permission from patient and then refer identified concerns to their own faith leader.

3. Chaplain referral. Place a referral to the hospital chaplain (preferably certified). Permission is typically not needed (i.e. do not ask the patient if they want to see the chaplain because you are then asking the patient for a self-assessment of their need and assuming they know what the role of the chaplain is, make a clear recommendation), it is similar to a referral to social services or a respiratory therapist as these specialists can better review and identify appropriate interventions (if any needed).

Source: Information from LaRocca-Pitts, M. (2009). In FACT, chaplains have a spiritual assessment tool. *American Journal of Pastoral Care and Health*, 3(2), 8–15.

PART II: SYMPTOMS

ANOREXIA-CACHEXIA SYNDROME

I. **Background information**
   A. Anorexia: Poor appetite or early satiety from a variety of etiologies; see mnemonic for potentially reversible causes:
   A: Aches (pain)
   N: Nausea
   O: Oral (candidiasis, mucositis, ulcerations, dentition, dysphagia)
   R: Reactive (neuropsychiatric: depression, anxiety, delirium)
   E: Evacuation (constipation)
   X: Xerostomia (dry mouth)
   I: Iatrogenic (radiation, chemotherapy, opioids)
   A: Acid-related (gastritis, peptic ulcer disease)
   - Terminal anorexia is part of the disease process, a natural part of life ending, and does not respond to additional calorie supplementation. Caregivers typically respond to the expected reduced oral intake with alarm and attempt to "push" calories.
     a. It is not starvation.
        i. Starving is due to a lack of needed calories (i.e., calories that the body can or is able to use).
     b. Force-feeding in this situation can lead to increased discomfort (nausea, bloating, and dyspnea) and can shorten life (aspiration, ascites, effusions, and heart failure).
     c. Allow patient to guide eating habits.
        i. Encourage family to show love without force-feeding in ways such as reading books, sharing stories, offering massages, and listening to favorite music.
   B. Cachexia: Involuntary weight loss (10% from premorbid weight) of primarily lean (skeletal) muscle mass (due to proteolysis) and fat (due to lipolysis).
     1. Primary cachexia is due to a metabolic syndrome resulting in increased catabolism.
        a. Proinflammatory cytokines involved include TNF-α, IL-1β and IL-6.
        b. Hormones involved include leptin and ghrelin.

      c. Anabolic abnormalities include decreased testosterone levels.

      d. Catabolic state is due to a chronic inflammatory response in the setting of cancer, heart failure, chronic obstructive pulmonary disease, AIDS, and chronic infections or autoimmune disorders.

   2. Secondary cachexia is due to decreased oral intake (anorexia) or malabsorption.

II. Evaluation

A. History includes inquiring about dietary habits, appetite, taste, weight loss, and a review of systems to identify etiologies of secondary cachexia.

B. Physician exam includes evaluating oropharynx (including ability to swallow), abdomen, and rectum.

- If necessary, labs would include a complete blood count, electrolytes, calcium, glucose, creatinine, liver function, albumin, prealbumin, and thyroid function.

III. Management

A. Treat cachexia based on underlying cause (disease or symptom identified).

- Consider dietitian evaluation and recommendations.

TABLE 6.1 Medications to Treat Anorexia or Cachexia

Medication Class	Drug/Dosing	Comments
Anabolic agents	Fluoxymesterone 20 mg/day Oxandrolone 10 mg PO two times per day	Last line agents as no overall benefit identified. Fluoxymesterone was found to be less effective than either dexamethasone or megestrol acetate. Oxandrolone has a theoretical benefit of increased lean mass but found to have decreased overall weight. Investigational: ghrelin or ghrelin analogues (can induce growth hormone).

(continues)

TABLE 6.1 (*continued*)

Medication Class	Drug/Dosing	Comments
Appetite stimulants (orexigenic)	Progestins (>6 weeks prognosis): Megastrol acetate 400 mg to 800 mg daily Corticosteroids (<6 weeks prognosis): Dexamethasone 4–8 mg PO q AM Cannabinoids: Dronabinol 2.5 mg PO twice per day up to 20 mg/day. Cyproheptadine up to 8 mg PO three times per day (for patients with carcinoid syndrome)	These medications may increase fatty tissue weight however no affect on increasing lean muscle mass. Megestrol acetate improves appetite, activity, and wellbeing and due to side effect profile preferred over dexamethasone. Side effects include peripheral edema, venous thromboembolism, and adrenal suppression with abrupt withdrawal. Corticosteroid benefits are lost within weeks and not recommended long term unless needed for underlying disease (such as chronic obstructive pulmonary disease) due to increased long-term side effects (immunosuppression, adrenal suppression, myopathy, osteoporosis, psychosis/delirium). Dronabinol does not offer any additional benefit to megestrol acetate alone. Side effects may limit use which include sedation, confusion, and drowsiness.
Anticatabolic—anticytokine agents	Eicosapentaenoic acid (omega-3 fatty acids EPA and DHA found in fish oil): 1.5 to 7.5 g/day. Thalidomide 200 mg/day (advanced pancreatic cancer) Melatonin 20 mg PO qPM	Investigational agents to modulate TNF-α (pentoxifylline, etanercept, and infliximab), IL-1β, IL-6, proteolysis-inducing factor, and lipid-mobilizing factor.
Prokinetic agents	Metoclopramide 10 mg PO before meals, at bedtime	1st choice if anorexia due to early satiety or gastroparesis present.
Antidepressants	Tetracyclics: mirtazapine 15 to 30 mg PO at bedtime	Side effects: weight gain, sedation.
Artificial nutrition and hydration		See Shared Decision Making, Allow patient's symptoms of hunger or thirst to guide decision making and consider time-limited trials in uncertain cases of benefit versus harm.

ASCITES, MALIGNANCY-RELATED

I. **Background information**
   A. Commonly associated with breast, colon, endometrial, gastric, ovarian (most common), pancreatic, and unknown primary cancers
   B. Symptoms associated with increasing ascites include pain, nausea, and dyspnea, and are due to increased hepatic venous pressure (due to mass effect from tumors), increased vascular permeability (due to effects of cytokines including VEGF), lymphatic obstruction, overactivation of the renin-angiotensin-aldosterone system, and/or neoplastic fluid production.

II. **Evaluation**
   A. Patients with suspected ascites
      1. Complete a thorough history (nausea, early satiety, dyspnea) and physical (abdominal distension/increased abdominal girth, shifting dullness, and fluid wave).
      2. Confirm ascites with an imaging study if indicated.
      3. Evaluate ascitic fluid (consider at a baseline cell count/differential, Gram stain/culture, cytology, protein, albumin, and other tests if indicated).
      4. Measure serum albumin at the same time to calculate the SAAG (serum albumin minus the ascitic fluid albumin).

III. **Management**
   A. Calculate SAAG
      1. If SAAG ≥1.1, then ascites is due to portal hypertension (mass effect from cancers, cirrhosis, heart failure, hepatic vein occlusion [Budd-Chiari syndrome])
         a. Lifestyle changes: Consider fluid and sodium restriction (balance with quality of life goals)
         b. Diuretics: Potassium sparing and loop diuretics
            i. Spironolactone 100–400 mg/day: takes up to 2 weeks for full diuretic effect
               (A) Consider amiloride if more rapid diuresis indicated
            ii. Furosemide 40–160 mg/day
            iii. Ideally should maintain ratio of 100 mg spironolactone to 40 mg furosemide while titrating
         c. Mechanical removal
            i. Serial paracentesis: If large volume (>5 liters), may benefit from colloid supplementation (6–8 grams of IV albumin/liter of fluid removed; utilize 5% albumin if hypovolemic, 25% if hypervolemic)
            ii. Consider transjugular intrahepatic portosystemic shunt (TIPS) if relatively good short-term prognosis
         d. Midodrine: 10 mg PO three times per day
            i. Can be considered especially if renal dysfunction present, if hypotensive, or as an alternative to IV albumin

2. If SAAG <1.1, then not due to portal hypertension; can be malignancy related, such as carcinomatosis, nephrotic syndrome, tuberculosis
   a. Mechanical removal
      i. Paracentesis: Can usually do high-volume paracentesis without significant hemodynamic compromise
      ii. Permanent indwelling catheter: For frequent small-volume drainage (at home) such as with a pigtail catheter (temporary, <1 month prognosis) or a tunneled catheter (long-term, prognosis >1 month, typically used for peritoneal dialysis)
      iii. Peritoneovenous shunt (LeVeen or Denver shunt): High rate of complications (acute pulmonary edema, DIC, venous thromboembolism, peritonitis, tumor seeding, encephalopathy, and shunt occlusion)
          (A) Reserve for patients with poor prognosis (1–3 months) and refractory ascites
          (B) Most useful for ovarian cancer in patients with normal renal function
          (C) Risk can be reduced if majority of ascitic fluid is drained prior to procedure
          (D) Advised 24-hour ICU monitoring of central venous pressure postprocedure
   b. Chemotherapy: Intraperitoneal or systemic
      i. Strongly consider for patients with ovarian cancer (along with surgical debulking)
   c. Consider diuretics
   d. Consider octreotide 200–600 micrograms/day SQ/IV
   e. Consider bevacizumab (Avastin) 5 mg/kg intraperitoneal q 4 weeks (small case studies: colorectal, breast, uterine, or ovarian cancer)

URINARY SYMPTOMS

I. Evaluation
   A. Incontinence: Based on history, examination (assess for fecal impaction), and urinalysis (assess for UTI)
      • Types
         a. Urge incontinence: From overactive bladder syndrome (detrusor muscle overactivity)
         b. Stress incontinence: From increased intra-abdominal pressure overcoming urethral sphincter function
         c. Mixed incontinence (urge plus stress): Most common in women
         d. Overflow incontinence: Most common in men, usually due to bladder outlet obstruction or detrusor muscle underactivity

TABLE 6.2 Incontinence Management Overview

Stress incontinence	Pelvic floor exercises Surgery Medications usually not helpful
Urge or Mixed incontinence	Avoid alcohol, carbonated drinks, coffee, or tea Advise frequent voluntary or prompted urination Consider medications

II. **Management**
  A. Medication
    1. Treatment utilizes anticholinergics with antimuscarinic activity
    2. Side effects include dry mouth, constipation, urinary retention, and possibly delirium
    3. Caution with dementia patients
       a. Oxybutynin
          i. Oxybutynin IR 2.5 mg PO two to three times per day (up to max 20 mg/day)
          ii. Oxybutynin ER 5 mg PO daily (up to max 30 mg/day)
          iii. Oxybutynin transdermal patch 3.9 mg/day q 3–4 days
          iv. Oxybutynin 10% gel (100 mg/g): Apply contents of 1 sachet once daily to dry, intact skin on the abdomen, upper arms/shoulder, or thighs
       b. Tolterodine IR 1–2 mg PO two times per day, tolterodine ER 2–4 mg PO daily
       c. Fesoterodine 4–8 mg PO daily (prodrug, metabolized to tolterodine)
       d. Trospium 20 mg PO daily (elderly) or two times per day (normal renal function), Trospium 60 mg ER PO daily (avoid if CrCl <30 mL/min)
  B. Management of Dysuria
     • Phenazopyridine 200 mg PO three times per day (up to 3 days, darkens urine, avoid if CrCl <50 mL/min)
       a. If chronic symptoms consider nortriptyline 10 mg PO at bedtime, titrate dose weekly as tolerated (side effects include dry mouth, urinary retention, sedation, orthostatic hypotension)
  C. Management of Bladder or ureteral spasms
     • Consider belladonna & opium suppositories #15 (belladonna extract 16.2 mg and opium 30 mg) or #16 (belladonna extract 16.2 mg and opium 60 mg): ½ to 1 PR daily to four times per day

D. Management of Urinary retention or overflow incontinence
1. Attempt to reduce or stop offending medications (phenyl-ephrine, tricyclic antidepressants, anticholinergics [such as scopolamine, glycopyrrolate, oxybutynin], antipsychotics, anti-histamines, opioids, and muscle relaxants)
   a. If due to opioids that need to be continued, consider meth-ylnaltrexone trial if intermittent catheterization not an option (limited evidence to support use)
   b. If due to BPH, consider terazosin, doxazosin, tamsulosin, and finasteride
2. Bethanechol (cholinergic; contracts the bladder but has lim-ited effectiveness): 10 mg PO single dose, then titrate hourly if needed
   a. Initial dose typically 10–50 mg three to four times per day with titration up to 100 mg four times per day
   b. Avoid using if GI/GU obstruction, seizure disorder, coronary artery disease, or parkinsonism present

ABDOMINAL BLOATING AND GAS

I. **Background information**
   A. Abdominal bloating from intestinal gas can lead to abdominal pain, belching, and flatulence.
II. **Evaluation**
   A. History
      • Take a thorough history for evidence of air swallowing (frequent swallowing of saliva, chewing gum, or smoking), carbonated beverages, and supine position after eating/drinking (more air enters into small intestine).
III. **Management**
   A. Lifestyle changes
      1. Trials of limiting carbonated beverages, and products contain-ing lactose, fructose, or sorbitol.
      2. Limiting certain foods such as bran, pork, legumes (alfalfa, beans, lentils, peanuts, and soy), and cruciferous vegetables (cauliflower, cabbage, and broccoli).
      3. Sitting fully upright after eating or drinking for at least 30 minutes, longer if able.
   B. Medication options
      1. Simethicone 40–360 mg po with meals, at bedtime, prn for bloating/flatulence.
      2. Alpha-galactosidase (Beano) 2–3 tablets or 10–15 drops per problem meal.
      3. Consider treatment for small intestinal bacterial overgrowth 7–10 days (e.g., amoxicillin-clavulanate 1500 mg/day with met-ronidazole 700 mg/day; alternative option is the more expensive rifaximin 800–1200 mg/day [nonabsorbable antibiotic]).

CONSTIPATION AND BOWEL OBSTRUCTION

I. **Background information**
   A. Constipation
      1. Syndrome consisting of infrequent or difficult defecation
      2. Because of individual differences, define according to each patient's baseline stool patterns
   B. Bowel obstruction
      • Can be due to mechanical etiologies (extrinsic or intraluminal occlusion) or functional etiologies (adynamic ileus)

II. **Evaluation**
   A. History
      1. Obtain history of bowel patterns, symptoms (colicky abdominal pain, nausea, vomiting, flatulence, urinary retention, distension, anorexia, delirium).
      2. Identify potential medications that can lead to constipation such as opioids, anticholinergics (antispasmodics and antidepressants), antipsychotics, iron, verapamil, 5HT3 antagonists (such as ondansetron), and diuretics.
   B. Examination
      1. Identify presence or absence of abdominal sounds.
      2. Palpate for masses (stool versus tumors) and tenderness.
      3. Rectal examination is needed to evaluate for fecal impaction, which will require manual disimpaction.
      4. Evaluate for hypercalcemia, hypokalemia, or hypothyroidism.
      5. A plain abdominal radiograph can help distinguish between constipation, obstruction, and ileus.

III. **Management**
   A. Constipation
      • Avoid bulk-forming agents (such as psyllium, methylcellulose, polycarbophil, and wheat dextrin) in most palliative patients due to impaired fluid intake and decreased mobility, and likelihood of being on opioids.
      Step 1: Combination of stool softener PLUS a stimulant
      Step 2: Add hyperosmolar or saline agents
      Step 3: Consider a prokinetic agent
      Step 4: Consider lubricants + enemas
      Step 5: Consider opioid antagonists

TABLE 6.3 Constipation Medications

Class	Medication/Dosage	Onset	Adverse Reactions
Stool softeners	Docusate Sodium 100 mg PO twice per day (up to 600 mg/day) Docusate calcium 240 mg PO daily	24–72 h	—
Hyperosmolar	Lactulose 10 g/15 mL 15–60 mL PO twice per day-three times per day or Sorbitol 70% 15–60 mL PO twice per day-three times per day or 25% 120 mL daily	24–48 h	Gas/flatulence, bloating, nausea. Lactulose and sorbitol's sweet taste can be unpleasant. Polyethylene glycol is tasteless and as a result may be preferred.
	Polyethylene glycol 17 g in 4–8 oz liquid daily (up to q 2 h prn until bowel movement) [Note: GoLYTELY brand includes electrolytes and given up to 4 liters]	24–96 h	
	Consider Lubiprostone 24 mcg PO twice per day (activates fluid secretion into intestines, 24 mcg dose used for adults with idiopathic constipation, 8 mcg dose used for women with IBS associated constipation)	24–48 h	Nausea, headache.
Saline	Magnesium hydroxide (Milk of magnesia) 15–30 mL daily-three times per day	4–8 h	Caution using magnesium products with renal or heart failure patients or if hypertension; avoid chronic use.
	Magnesium citrate 240 mL daily	0.5–3 h	
Stimulants	Prune juice 120–240 mL PO daily-twice per day	6–12 h	Cramping, colic. Avoid in bowel obstruction.
	Senna 1–4 tabs up to twice daily	6–12 h	
	Bisacodyl 5mg 1–3 PO up to twice daily or 10 mg PR daily	PO or 15–60 min PR	
Lubricants	Glycerin 1 PR daily	15–60 min	Irritant
	Mineral Oil 10–30 mL PO daily or 133 mL PR daily	6–8 h	Caution if aspiration risk (pneumonitis), avoid if using docusate due to increased mineral oil absorption.

(continues)

TABLE 6.3 (*continued*)

Class	Medication/Dosage	Onset	Adverse Reactions
Enemas	Sodium phosphate 1 PR daily Warm "tap" water 1 PR daily – twice per day Soap suds 1 PR daily Mineral oil 1 PR daily	2–20 min 2–15 min	Caution with sodium phosphate in renal or heart failure. Avoid chronic use.
Prokinetics	Metoclopramide 10–20 mg PO q 6 h Bethanechol 25 mg PO four times per day		Avoid in complete bowel obstruction. Limited evidence to support bethanechol use.
Opioid antagonists	Naloxone up to 4 mg PO three times per day Methylnatrexone sq q 24–48 h 38–61 kg 8 mg 62–114 kg 12 mg <38 kg or >114 kg 0.15 mg/kg (half dose if creatinine clearance <30 mL/min)	<2 h	Naloxone can have some degree of opioid reversal symptoms due to minimal systemic absorption; start low dose and titrate as tolerated. Methylnatrexone can increase abdominal pain, flatulence, nausea, diarrhea, and hyperhidrosis.

B. Bowel obstruction
- Nonoperative acute management includes rapid decompression via nasogastric suction and fluid resuscitation.
  a. Advise surgical assessment for determining need for operative management if indicated (generally if prognosis >2 months).
     i. If long-term decompression needed, advise venting gastrostomy (i.e., PEG)
        (A) Avoid if portal hypertension, large ascites, high bleeding risk, and caution if multiple prior surgeries or carcinomatosis.
     ii. Consider gastrointestinal assessment to evaluate if stenting might be beneficial.
     iii. Consider TPN if death might be due to starvation (i.e., patient is clearly hungry and thirsty, not in a terminal cachexia state, and consistent with goals of care) rather than end-stage tumor progression (in which risks are significantly increased).
     iv. Ensure adequate opioid pain control.

TABLE 6.4 Bowel Obstruction Medications

Class	Medication	Adverse Reactions
Anticholinergics (decrease GI secretions)	Glycopyrrolate 0.1–0.2 mg IV/SQ q 6 h up to 0.8 mg/day Scopolamine 40–120 mg/day continuous SQ infusion or 1.5 mg transdermal patch	Urinary retention, dry mouth, constipation, nausea Scopolamine hydrobromide crosses the blood–brain barrier and can potentiate delirium
Inhibitory hormone (decrease secretions)	Octreotide 200–900 mcg/day via continuous SC/IV infusion or 50–100 mcg SQ q 8 h and titrate up to 900 mcg/day	Headache, cramps, nausea, constipation, gallstones/ hyperbilirubinemia, fluctuating glucose levels
Antiemetics	Haloperidol 5–20 mg/day IV/SQ	Tardive dyskinesia, drowsiness, caution QT prolongation with haloperidol and balance risks/ benefits.
	Dexamethasone 4–12 mg IV/SQ daily	Anxiety, hyperglycemia, edema. Avoid if surgery planned
Example mixture	Combine as appropriate a combination of the above in 60–100 mL normal saline and infuse IV or SQ over 24 h. Other agents to consider in mix: diphenhydramine 25–100 mg metoclopramide 40–120 mg if partial SBO and if no cramping.	Consider mixing an anti- cholinergic + octreotide + antiemetic

DIARRHEA

I. Background information

A. Passage of more than 3 stools in 24 hours
   - Acute if <2 weeks, persistent if 2–4 weeks, chronic if >4 weeks in duration

II. Evaluation

A. Acute diarrhea
   - If severe and needed after appropriate history and physical (i.e., hypovolemic, fevers, pain, bleeding), consider evaluating with stool culture, stool leukocytes (consider antibiotics if positive or fevers while awaiting stool culture), and stool for *C. difficile*. Treat reversible causes identified.

B. Chronic diarrhea
- If appropriate after history and physical (rule out bowel obstruction or fecal impaction), obtain screening labs.
  a. Baseline evaluation may include CBC (leukocytosis, eosinophilia), electrolytes, renal and liver function, thyroid function, and protein levels.
  b. To classify diarrhea as watery (secretory or osmotic), inflammatory, or fatty, obtain the following as appropriate:
     i. Calculate stool osmolal gap
        (A) [Stool Osm] − 2([Stool Na+] + [Stool K+])
        (B) If >125 mOsm/kg, then osmotic diarrhea (due to laxatives for example)
        (C) If <50 mOsm/kg, then secretory (usually due to a stimulant such as with tumor syndromes like carcinoid or chronic infection; may improve with fasting)
     ii. Stool pH, if <5.6, then carbohydrate malabsorption
     iii. Fecal occult blood: If positive, consider inflammatory bowel disease, neoplasm, and celiac sprue
     iv. Stool leukocytes: If positive, suggests inflammatory diarrhea
     v. Stool fat concentration: If >8% (or if >14 grams/24 hours), consider pancreatic exocrine insufficiency
     vi. Other? Laxative screening (including iatrogenic due to sorbitol base in many elixirs), enteroscopy, colonoscopy (radiation-induced?), tumor syndrome (5-HIAA [carcinoid syndrome], gastrin [gastrinoma/Zollinger-Ellison], vasoactive intestinal peptide [VIPoma])

III. **Management**
A. Hydration: Orally via glucose/electrolyte solutions or IV lactated ringers; consider bulk-forming agents if tolerated (psyllium, methylcellulose).
B. Opiates are most effective.
   1. Loperamide (Imodium)
      a. Acute: 4 mg PO single dose, then 2 mg after each unformed stool up to 16 mg/day. Avoid if due to infection such as *C. difficile*.
      b. Chronic: Initially treat as above, then maintain with 2 mg PO twice daily.
      c. Does not cross the blood–brain barrier
      d. Has been used up to 32 mg/day
   2. Less effective or increased side effect alternatives include diphenoxylate/atropine (lomotil 2.5 mg/0.025 mg up to 2 tabs PO q 6 h), codeine (10–60 mg PO q 4 h), or tincture of opium (0.3–1 mL PO q 6 h prn)

3. Radiation-induced diarrhea
   a. Medication: Cholestyramine (4 g PO three times per day), sulfasalazine (500 mg PO twice daily), aspirin (325 mg PO up to q 4 h) and corticosteroids
   b. Consider TPN and surgical evaluation for refractory cases.
4. Chemotherapy-induced, dumping syndrome, or carcinoid: Octreotide 100 microgram SQ twice daily up to 600 micrograms/day SQ/IV (intermittent or continuous infusion)
   a. Reduce octreotide over several days to lowest effective dose.
5. Other options: bismuth subsalicylate, probiotics, clonidine (for opioid withdrawal or diabetic diarrhea)

DYSPEPSIA AND GASTROESOPHAGEAL REFLUX DISEASE (GERD)

I. Background information
A. Dyspepsia
   - Chronic or recurrent discomfort in the upper abdomen
B. GERD
   - Dyspeptic symptoms predominantly consisting of heartburn due to reflux into the esophagus (with or without regurgitation to the oropharynx)

II. Evaluation
A. Consider EGD if clinically appropriate and evaluation for *H. pylori* for patients with alarm symptoms or those older than 55 years (consider if prognosis >3–6 months).
   - Alarm symptoms: weight loss, progressive dysphagia, recurrent vomiting, evidence of gastrointestinal bleeding, or family history of cancer

III. Management
A. Dietary and lifestyle changes
   1. Elevate head of bed 4–8 inches with blocks or phone books.
   2. Avoid eating just before lying down.
   3. Avoid caffeine and alcohol/red wine. Less evidence for limiting fatty foods, chocolate, peppermint, sodas, orange juice (may have more to do with too large a size of meal than the food itself as injury is primarily due to endogenous acid production refluxing into esophagus).
   4. Avoid tight-fitting clothes.
   5. Avoid smoking.
   6. Consider chewing gum (increased salivation neutralizes acid).
B. H2-receptor antagonists: famotidine, ranitidine, and nizatidine
   1. Can consider cimetidine, however should avoid in elderly due to CNS toxicity and multiple drug interactions.
   2. Caution with antihistamines in general in elderly patients prone to delirium (use lower doses as appropriate for age and renal function).

C. Proton pump inhibitor therapy: omeprazole, lansoprazole, rabeprazole, pantoprazole, esomeprazole, and dexlansoprazole
D. *H. pylori* testing: Advised if prognosis generally greater than 3–6 months
  • Serology easiest, then consider breath testing or stool for antigen testing if needed (if not taking PPI and no active bleeding)
E. Prokinetic therapy
  1. Metoclopramide 5–10 mg PO before meals/at bedtime (multiple side effects, generally avoid if possible)
  2. Bethanechol 25 mg PO 1 hour before meals and at bedtime (cholinergic)
F. Other therapy
  1. Sucralfate 1 g PO before meals/at bedtime
  2. Misoprostol 100–200 before meals/at bedtime (with proton pump inhibitor/especially if NSAIDs required)
  3. Aluminum hydroxide plus magnesium hydroxide (Maalox plus) 15–30 mL PO up to q 2 hours (consider mixing with 5 mL of viscous 2% lidocaine or 20% benzocaine)

OROPHARYNX: DYSPHAGIA, MUCOSITIS, XEROSTOMIA, AND HALITOSIS

I. **Background information**
  A. Dysphagia
    • Difficulty swallowing
      a. If solid food dysphagia developed prior to liquid dysphagia, then likely due to mechanical obstruction (such as from head and neck cancers, esophageal cancer, esophagitis, GERD, achalasia, scleroderma, NSAIDs, and potassium chloride)
      b. If simultaneously developed solid and liquid dysphagia, then likely due to neuromuscular disorders (such as stroke, ALS, Parkinson's disease, multiple sclerosis, and myasthenia gravis)
      c. Could be from odynophagia (pain with swallowing), dry mouth, periodontal disease, and mucosal damage
  B. Mucositis
    1. Radiation induced with mucosal erythema and pseudomembranous reaction up to deep ulcers
    2. Stomatitis from chemotherapy with painless or painful ulcers
      a. Due to damage of the mucosal barrier from any etiology
    3. Typically develops in those with underlying poor oral hygiene or pre-chemo or radiation periodontal disease
  C. Xerostomia
    • Dry mouth
      a. Noted in up to 40% of hospice patients; most common in cancer patients

b. Can be due to infection (viral/fungal), drugs (anticholinergics, antihistamines, phenothiazines, antidepressants, opioids, beta-blockers, diuretics, anticonvulsants, and antipsychotics), dehydration, mucositis, and mouth breathing

D. Halitosis
- Bad breath mostly (80–90%) originates from bacteria between the teeth and the posterior part of the tongue, possibly from postnasal drip.
  a. Halitosis is worse when the mouth is dry.
  b. Next most common source is the nasal passages, then tonsils, and finally more systemic etiologies (pulmonary infections, renal failure, liver failure, smoking, and various cancers).

II. Evaluation

A. Focused history and physical
  1. Consider speech therapy evaluation if dysphagia present.
  2. Consider invasive testing if appropriate (modified barium swallow, upper endoscopy).
  3. Identify common lesions.
    a. Candidiasis starts with painless white flecks or patches that adhere firmly but can be scraped off with underlying mucosal bleeding.
    b. HSV starts with vesicles that rupture to form irregularly bordered small (5 mm) ulcers with erythematous margin and gray center. Gingiva is painful, swollen, and may bleed. Lip lesions may crust over.
    c. Aphthous stomatitis (cancer sores) lacks a vesicular stage and has painful lesions from 1–15 mm located on the soft mucosa (not on gingiva or hard palate).

B. Grading mucositis
  - National Cancer Institute Common Toxicity Criteria v3.0:
    a. Mucosal erythema (normal diet, minimal symptoms)
    b. Patchy ulcers or pseudomembranes (tolerates modified diet)
    c. Confluent ulcers or pseudomembranes, easy bleeding (unable to eat or drink adequately)
    d. Tissue necrosis, spontaneous bleeding (life-threatening)

III. Management

A. Dysphagia
  - Depends on etiology
    a. If from obstructive etiology, consider stenting, radiation, surgery, or less invasive options if possible (speech therapy recommendations advised).
    b. Treat identified infections (candidiasis, HSV).

B. Mucositis
1. Dietary
   a. Soft, bland diet (avoid crackers, granola, chips, pretzels; use cooked pasta, cooked cereals, boiled vegetables, mashed potatoes, and soft fruits).
   b. Avoid spicy or fried foods and citrus drinks (choose fruit nectars instead).
2. Oral adjustments
   a. Consider short-term denture removal until healed.
   b. Oral hygiene up to every 2 hours.
3. Consider topical honey (even alongside initial radiation therapy to help reduce severity)
4. Medication
   a. Viscous lidocaine (Xylocaine) 2%: Swish and spit before meals
   b. Sucralfate suspension: 5 mL swish 3–4 ×/day
   c. Mouthwash mixture (1:1:1): Diphenhydramine, viscous lidocaine (Xylocaine) 2%, and Maalox (aluminum hydroxide plus magnesium hydroxide, or Kaopectate).
   d. Morphine mouthwash: 15 mL of 0.2% morphine solution (2000 mg morphine chlorhydrate diluted in 1000 mL of water)
      i. Rinse/hold in mouth and spit out q 3 h as needed.
   e. Candidiasis: Clotrimazole 10 mg troches dissolved 5 ×/day for 7–14 days, fluconazole 100–200 mg PO daily for 7–14 days, or nystatin suspension (with aggressive oral care) 5 mL swish/swallow 4 ×/day (ideally should be held in mouth for several minutes) for 7–14 days
   f. HSV
      i. Acyclovir 200 mg po 5 ×/day (or 400 mg PO three times per day) for 7–10 days.
      ii. Famciclovir 500 mg PO twice daily for 7 days.
      iii. Valacyclovir 100 mg PO twice daily for 10 days.
      iv. Above medications require adjustments for renal function.
   g. If aphthous ulcer: Triamcinolone oral rinse 5 mL after meals/ at bedtime (60 mL Kenalog–40 plus 200 mL of NS)
C. Xerostomia
1. Increase saliva production
   a. Chewing sugar-free non-cinnamon/mint gum, sucking on sugar-free lemon drops, eating pineapple chunks or ice chips, drinking water, coating mouth with flavored yogurt, eating frozen juice, using a moist sponge stick
   b. Avoid lemon or glycerine swabs (increased dryness can result)
2. For dry lips, utilize petroleum-based lip balm
3. Saliva substitutes q 1–2 hours

4. Pilocarpine 5–10 mg PO three times per day (caution if glaucoma, cardiac history, and if diaphoresis)
5. Adjust causative medications if possible
D. Halitosis
   1. Optimize oral hygiene.
      a. Regular brushing (soft bristles with gel toothpaste), flossing (including posterior surface of the most distal tooth), brushing the posterior portion of the tongue, and gargling with an alcohol-free mouth rinse.
   2. Nasal sinus rinses.
   3. If due to oral bleeding, consider topical thrombin to bleeding areas or tranexamic acid.
   4. Thick mucus: Sodium bicarbonate mouthwash (10 mL sodium bicarbonate to 1 L of NS).
   5. Hardened debris: Hydrogen peroxide mouthwash (5 mL 3% hydrogen peroxide + 20 mL water, prepared just before each use. Caution patients may feel a burning sensation).

NAUSEA AND VOMITING

I. **Background information**
   A. Nausea
      • Unpleasant sensation near the region of the stomach with the feeling of the need to vomit
   B. Emesis (vomiting)
      1. Forceful oral expulsion of the gastric contents (via reflexive abdominal wall contractions, pylorus/antrum contractions, decreased lower esophageal sphincter pressure, esophageal dilation, and reverse peristalsis)
         a. Retching includes most of the muscular events of vomiting, but without the expulsion of gastric contents.
      2. Vomiting center
         a. The sensation and muscular events that lead up to emesis are neurologically controlled by the vomiting center (lateral reticular formation of the medulla), which includes multiple receptors that can be targeted by specific interventions (D2-dopamine, 5-HT3-serotonin, M-muscarinic/acetylcholine, H1-histamine, NK1-neurokinin)
         b. The vomiting center is the final common pathway of emesis with signals arriving from four general sources:
            i. Cerebral cortex: Elevated intracranial pressure, pain, migraines, emotional input such as anticipation, anxiety, or prior memories
            ii. Vestibular system (middle ear): Labyrinthitis, motion sickness (kinetosis), and vertigo; receptors include histamine and acetylcholine

      iii. GI tract: gastric distension, gag reflex, GERD, mechanical obstruction, and GI tract irritation from any etiology such as infections, radiation, chemotherapy, toxins, and medications
         (A) Receptors include peripheral mechano-/chemoreceptors, dopamine, and serotonin.
      iv. Chemoreceptor trigger zone (CTZ): Located on the floor of the fourth ventricle, an area without a true blood–brain barrier, which is exposed to the systemic circulation
         (A) Can be triggered by uremia, hypercalcemia, pregnancy, medications (opioids, digoxin, antibiotics, chemotherapy, and theophylline), hyperglycemia, hypocortisolism, and hyponatremia.
         (B) Receptors include dopamine, serotonin, acetylcholine, and opioid (Mu).

II. Evaluation

  A. "A-VOMIT"
    A: Anxiety/anticipatory
    V: Vestibular
    O: Obstructive, constipation
    M: Medications/metabolic
    I: Inflammation (infection: GI or GU tract, peptic ulcers)/increased intracranial pressure
    T: Toxins
  B. Tip: Generally large-volume emesis is from gastric outflow obstruction; small volume from gastric stasis

III. Management

  A. If tolerating oral intake, consider sips of clear liquids (apple juice, broth, ginger ale, gelatin, or ginger tea), world health organization oral rehydration solutions, and small bites of bland foods (mashed potatoes, applesauce, crackers, or toast)
  B. Consider acupuncture or vitamin B6 25 mg PO three times per day as appropriate (e.g., for pregnant patients with mild symptoms)
  C. Medications
    • Select an initial medication that targets the appropriate receptors after the likely etiology is identified or during workup and titrate as needed.
     a. If more than one agent required, use an agent that targets another receptor after the first agent has been titrated.
     b. Antiemetics can be scheduled if nausea/vomiting is persistent or as needed if intermittent.

TABLE 6.5 Nausea Management Medications

Drug	Dosage	Notes
Prokinetics		
Metoclopramide (Reglan)	5–15 mg PO/SQ/IV q 6–8 h	Also has dopamine antagonist activity
Anticholinergics		
Scopolamine	1.5-mg transdermal patch q 3 days or 0.3–0.6 mg IM/IV/SQ q 6 h	–
Antihistamines		
Hydroxyzine (Atarax/Vistaril)	25–100 mg PO/IM q 4–6 h	–
Dimenhydrinate (Dramamine)	50–100 mg PO/IM/IV q 4–6 h	–
Diphenhydramine (Benadryl)	25–50 mg PO/IM/IV q 4–6 h	–
Moclizine (Antivert)	25–50 mg PO q 6 h	–
Promethazine (Phenergan)	12.5–25 mg PO/IM/IV q 4–6 h; 25 mg PR q 6 hours	Use central line if IV used to reduce risk of extravasation-related severe tissue injury
Dopamine Antagonists		
Haloperidol	0.5–5 mg PO q 6–8 h 2 mg IV/SQ q 8 h	Caution with elderly dementia patients
Chlorpromazine (Thorazine)	10–25 mg PO q 4–6 h 25–50 mg IM q 4 h	Switch IM to PO route as soon as possible Caution with elderly dementia patients
Droperidol (Inapsine)	0.625–1.25 mg IM/IV q 4 h	Caution due to increased QT risk Caution with elderly dementia patients
Olanzapine	2.5–7.5 mg PO/ODT at bedtime	Caution with elderly dementia patients
Prochlorperazine maleate (Compazine)	5–10 mg PO q 6 h 25 mg PR q 12 h	Caution with elderly dementia patients
Serotonin 5HT3 Antagonists		
Dolasetron (Anzemet)	12.5 mg IV daily prn N/V 100 mg PO 1 h pre-chemo or 2 h pre-surgery	IV should no longer used pre-chemo due to increased QT risk Headache and constipation are common side effects

(continues)

TABLE 6.5 (*continued*)

Drug	Dosage	Notes
Serotonin 5HT3 Antagonists (*continued*)		
Ondansetron (Zofran)	4–8 mg PO/IM/IV q 4–8 h	Differing pre-chemo and pre-radiation dosage regimens available as well Caution due to increased QT risk; note: headache and constipation are common side effects
Granisetron (Kytril)	1 mg PO q 12 h 10 mcg/kg IV q 12 hours Seven-day transdermal patch available for chemotherapy-induced nausea/vomiting (patients receiving daily chemotherapy for up to 5 days)	Typically given once for chemo/XRT/postop nausea/vomiting prevention Caution due to increased QT risk Headache and constipation are common side effects
Palonosetron	0.25 mg IV given 30 min prior to chemo	Not effective at stopping N/V once it occurs Caution due to increased QT risk; note: headache and constipation are common side effects
Steroids		
Dexamethasone	6–10 mg PO/SQ/IM/IV single dose then maintain 4–20 mg PO/IM/IV qam	Prednisone 5 mg = dexamethasone 0.75 mg
Cannabinoids		
Dronabinol	5–10 mg PO q 6–8 h	Very high delirium risk limits usefulness in most palliative care patients
Benzodiazepines		
Lorazepam	0.5–2 mg PO/IM/IV q 4–6 h	–
Diazepam	2–10 mg PO/IM/IV q 4–6 h	–
Neurokinin 1 Antagonists		
Aprepitant (Emend)	40 mg PO single dose prior to anesthesia for postop nausea/vomiting prevention 125 mg PO single dose 1 hour prior to moderate–high emetogenic chemo, then 80 mg qam on days 2 and 3 (along with corticosteroid and 5-HT3 antagonist)	–
Other		
Trimethobenzamide (Tigan)	300 mg PO q 6 hours (200 mg IM q 6 hours)	–

7 ■ NEUROPSYCHIATRIC

ANXIETY

I. **Background information**
  A. State of helplessness or apprehension whose source is not easily identified
     1. Different from fears (or phobias) whose source is clearly definable.
     2. Worry is often a component of both and is a concern about a real or imagined threat.
     3. Akathisia is a state of restlessness, such as an inability to sit still.
II. **Evaluation**
  A. Identify etiology if possible.
     • Generally can be broken down into 4 categories:
        a. Physical (disease-related symptoms, medications)
        b. Psychological (depression, delirium)
        c. Social (financial, being a burden, welfare of surviving family)
        d. Spiritual (existential)
  B. If needed after completing a thorough history, obtain relevant confirmatory studies (electrolytes, calcium, thyroid function tests, etc.)
  C. Often associated with depression (up to 60%) and should be assessed and treated alongside anxiety
     • Generalized anxiety disorder (GAD) is characterized as feeling anxious with an inability to control worry for at least 6 months
        a. Associated with decreased functional status due to at least 3 of the following: restlessness, fatigue, difficulty concentrating, irritability, muscle tension, and insomnia.
        b. It is not GAD if a specific fear or if another cause is identified.

TABLE 7.1 Anxiety-Causing Fears

Specific Fear	Potential Diagnosis
Fear of panic	Panic disorder
Fear of embarrassment	Social phobia
Fear of contamination	Obsessive-compulsive disorder
Fear of being away from family	Separation-anxiety disorder
Fear of gaining weight	Anorexia nervosa
Fear of serious illness (when none present)	Hypochondria

TABLE 7.2 Disease- and Medication-Related Causes of Anxiety

Disease States	Medications
Uncontrolled pain	Drug withdrawal syndromes (barbiturates, benzodiazepines, opioids, alcohol)
Hypoxia	Anticholinergics (benztropine, diphenhydramine, oxybutynin, tricyclics)
Sepsis	
Delirium	Dopaminergics (bromocriptine, levodopa, metoclopramide)
Hypoglycemia	
Hypocalcemia	Stimulants (aminophylline, caffeine, cocaine, methylphenidate, theophylline)
Bleeding/bruising	
Venous thromboembolism	Sympathomimetics (ephedrine, pseudoephedrine)
Dyspnea	
Hormone-secreting tumors	Corticosteroids
Hyperthyroidism	Beta-agonists
	Anti-psychotics

III. Management

A. Cognitive interventions
   1. Cognitive behavioral therapy: Utilize prior to medical interventions or concurrently after medication titration has been completed.
   2. Relaxation techniques such as breathing exercises and progressive muscle relaxation
   3. Massage therapy, pet therapy, aromatherapy, relaxing conversations, quiet environment, softly lit surroundings
B. Medical interventions
   1. Address concrete fears prior to medicating.
      a. Ask patient, "What worries you the most?"
      b. Provide time for the patient to ventilate all of his or her worries.
      c. Have appropriate professionals help manage identified worries (physician, social worker, pharmacist, chaplain).
      d. Adjust or manage contributing medical conditions or medications.
   2. If prognosis <1 month:
      a. Utilize rapid-acting interventions such as benzodiazepines.
   3. If prognosis >1 month:
      a. Utilize benzodiazepines short-term while long-term agents are initiated and titrated starting with Selective Serotonin Reuptake Inhibitors (SSRIs).

TABLE 7.3 Pharmacological Interventions for Anxiety

Benzodiazepines

Short acting
- Alprazolam 0.25–2 mg PO/SL q 6–8 h (PO peaks in 1–2 h; Use short term as needed due to short half life or pre-procedural for example)
- For refractory anxiety: midazolam 0.2 mg/kg bolus IV/SQ ×1 (or 0.1 mg/kg bolus q 30 min ×2), then 0.5–5 mg/h (start 25% of loading dose/h). IV onset in 1–5 minutes, Peak (IM): 30–60 min. T ½ 1–4 hours

Medium acting
- Lorazepam 0.5–2 mg PO/SL/IV/IM q 6–8 h. IV onset in 5–20 min, oral peak 2 h
- Oxazepam 10–30 mg three to four times per day (peak 2–4 hours)
- Temazepam 7.5–30 mg PO at bedtime (Used primarily for insomnia, peak 2–3 hours)

Long acting
- Clonazepam 0.25–0.5 mg PO q 8–12 h (onset 20–60 min, peaks in 1–3 h)
- Diazepam 2–10 mg PO/SL/PR/IV two to four times per day (onset with rapid peak in 15–45 min, active metabolites increases potential for oversedation with routine dosing. T ½ of metabolite 50–100 hours)

SSRIs

Useful for chronic anxiety states. Consider if depression component or prognosis >1 month. Less sedation & dry mouth than TCAs, decreased libido, need to taper off, consider ½ dose for frail elderly patients.

- Citalopram/Escitalopram 10–20 mg PO daily (less activating than fluoxetine).
- Fluoxetine 10–40 mg PO daily (potentially activating and can result in increased risk of insomnia and worsening of anxiety, no need to taper off)
- Paroxetine 10–50 mg PO daily (more sedating, weight gain, sexual side effects)
- Sertraline 50–200 mg PO daily (less activating than fluoxetine)

Tricyclic antidepressants

Useful for chronic anxiety states. Consider if depression component or prognosis >1 month. Consider also if insomnia or neuropathic pain present.

- Amitriptyline 10–150 mg at bedtime (metabolized to nortriptyline)
- Clomipramine 25–100 mg PO daily (obsessive compulsive disorder)
- Desipramine 10–150 mg PO at bedtime (less effects vs. imipramine)
- Imipramine 75–150 mg PO at bedtime (metabolized to desipramine)
- Nortriptyline 10–75 mg PO at bedtime (less side effects vs. amitriptyline)
- Doxepin 10–50 mg PO at bedtime (sedating)

Neuroleptics

First line if due to delirium or paranoia. Consider using as an adjuvant for severe anxiety or if agitation present.

- Chlorpromazine 10–25 mg PO/IV/SQ q 2–4 h prn. Infusion 10 mg/h titrating by 5–10 mg/h q 4 h
- Haloperidol 0.5–5 mg PO/SL/SQ/IV twice per day and q 4 h prn (PO peaks in 3–6 h)
- Olanzapine 5–12.5 mg PO/SL at bedtime (has been used in combination with fluoxetine)
- Quetiapine 50–300 mg PO divided qhs to two times per day (has been used for GAD, also daily dosing for depression, two times per day dosing for delirium)
- Risperidone 1–6 mg PO/SL divided daily to two times per day (titrate with twice daily dosing, then can change to daily once maintenance dose achieved)

(continues)

TABLE 7.3 (*continued*)

Other
• Buspirone 5–20 mg PO two to three times per day (Use as adjuvant to SSRIs, takes 3–4 weeks for full effect)
• Mirtazapine 7.5–45 mg PO at bedtime (lower doses more sedating)
• Propranolol 30–120 mg PO divided two to three times per day (Useful for akathisia)
• Venlafaxine XR 37.5–225 mg PO daily (useful for concomitant neuropathic pain, relief in 1–2 weeks)

Terminal Anxiety/Agitation
Utilize a sedation scale for monitoring and titration if nursing protocol utilized.
• Thiopental 5–7 mg/kg IV ×1, then 20–180 mg/h (pentobarbital active metabolite via liver metabolism)
• Pentobarbital 2–3 mg/kg IV ×1, then 1 mg/kg/h and titrate to maintain sedation (avoid SQ use)
• Phenobarbital 200 mg IV/SQ ×1 (or 10 mg/kg IV/SQ ×1), then 10–25 mg/h titrate up to 100 mg/h
• Propofol 20–50 mg ×1, then 10 mg/h and increase by 10 mg/h q 15 min as needed. (1 mg/kg/h with 15 minute titration of 0.5 mg/kg/h). Caution of >24–48 h usage (pancreatitis risk due to hypertriglyceridemia; caution with elevated pCO_2)

DELIRIUM

I. **Background information**
   A. Acute onset of diminished consciousness (inattention) and altered cognition (decreased ability to process information) that fluctuates over time
      1. Can have hypoactive or hyperactive features and is usually worse at night ("sundowning")
      2. Can last days to months
      3. Hallucinations common (as opposed to depression or dementia)
II. **Risk factors**

TABLE 7.4 Risk Factors for Delirium

Altered routines	Medications (polypharmacy)	Postoperative state
Constipation	Pain	Sensory impairments
Dementia	Poor functional status	(auditory, visual)
Elderly	(immobility, restraints,	Stroke
Insomnia	indwelling catheters,	
Malignancy	deconditioning)	

III. Evaluation

A. Complete a focused history and physical to help identify contributing etiologies and workup, and treat as appropriate for the patient's goals of care. Screening tools available include the confusion assessment method.

TABLE 7.5 Confusion Assessment Method (CAM) Delirium Screening

Mandatory Features	Either Feature
Acute, fluctuating AND Inattention (difficulty focusing, easily distractible)	Incoherent Altered consciousness (vigilant, lethargic, stuporous, or comatose)

Source: Adapted from Inouye, S. K., van Dyck, C. H., Alessi, C. A., Balkin, S., Siegal, A. P., & Horwitz, R. I. (1990). Clarifying confusion: the confusion assessment method. A new method for detection of delirium. *Annals of Internal Medicine,* 113(12), 941–948.

B. For ICU screening tools CAM-ICU or Intensive care delirium screening checklist (ICDSC) see www.icudelirium.org.
C. If delirium confirmed then identify etiologies.

TABLE 7.6 Common Etiologies ("DELIRIUM" Mnemonic)

'DELIRIUM' Mnemonic (etiologies)
Drugs (sedatives, opioids, steroids)
Electrolytes/metabolic (ca, glucose, thyroid)
Lack of drug (withdrawal from medications or from not enough, such as inadequate pain relief), water (dehydration), oxygen
Infection
Reduced sensory input (visual, hearing), Retention of feces (constipation)
Intracranial (stroke, seizure)
Urinary (infection, retention)
Myocardial (ischemia)

IV. Management

TABLE 7.7 Nonpharmacologic Interventions for Delirium

• Avoid dehydration (IVFs if indicated). • Reorient patient every shift. • Stimulate cognition. • Provide hearing aids/glasses. • Remove catheters/lines/restraints. • Decrease lights/sounds at night (open window coverings/keep lights on during the day). • Familiar faces around room. • Utilize sitters when possible.	• Educate families that fluctuations are expected and can be worse at night. • Encourage to be present as much as possible (if a calming influence to patient). • Confirm goals of care and prepare family for fluctuating course over time. • Discuss with families the risks and benefits of a time-limited trial of IV hydration to treat delirium at the end-of-life as in some patients may improve energy and mental status in the final days of life.

TABLE 7.8 Pharmacologic Interventions for Delirium

Medication (antipsychotics have been associated with increased mortality in the elderly population; discuss risks and benefits with surrogates)	Dosing (prn Delirium and Maintenance)	Comments
Chlorpromazine	PRN: 10–200 mg PO q 6 h or 25 mg IV 1 h (max 800 mg/24 hours). Schedule routine q 6–12 h (or via infusion).	Utilize for agitated delirium. More sedating than haloperidol.
Haloperidol	PRN: 0.5–1 mg PO/SL/SL/IV/SQ q 1 h (max 100 mg/24 h). Schedule routine q 6–12 h.	First-line agent. If high EPS risk consider adding benztropine. Avoid with Parkinson's symptoms and Lewy Body Dementia. Can be used for hypoactive delirium.
Olanzapine	PRN: 1.25–5 mg PO/ODT q 6 h (max 20 mg/24 hours). Schedule routine nightly.	–
Quetiapine	PRN: 12.5–50 mg q 2 hours (max 300 mg/24 h). Schedule routine nightly to twice daily.	Least anti-dopaminergic (Drug of choice for Parkinson's and Lewy-Body Dementia)
Risperidone	PRN: 0.25–1 mg PO/ODT q 1 h (max 6 mg/24 h). Schedule routine nightly to twice daily.	Least sedating of atypical antipsychotics. Can be used for hypoactive delirium.
Lorazepam	PRN: 0.5–2 mg PO/SL q 60 min SQ/IV q 30 min prn. Schedule routine q 6 h.	Use for terminal delirium, alcohol withdrawal, or agitation. Can paradoxically worsen delirium. Benzodiazepines do not clear sensorium or improve cognition.
Methylphenidate	2.5–5 mg PO qam and q noon.	Consider utilizing as an adjuvant to haloperidol or risperidone for hypoactive delirium.

A. Sedation for refractory symptoms
  1. Discuss with surrogates risks and benefits.
      a. Risks include unconsciousness that may need to be maintained indefinitely.
      b. Benefits include relief of refractory symptoms.
      c. Ensure documentation that all parties (healthcare team and patient/surrogates) are in agreement.
  2. Patients should be terminal (prognosis measured in days).
  3. All other treatments attempted (consider second opinion), resuscitation and artificial nutrition interventions discussed and addressed, and if appropriate, psychiatric/spiritual assessments completed (i.e., to confirm symptoms are not as a result of emotional or existential suffering)
  4. Should be titrated to lowest dose needed for symptom control

TABLE 7.9 Sedation for Refractory Symptoms

Drug	Dose	Comments
Midazolam	0.2 mg/kg bolus IV/SQ single dose (or 0.1 mg/kg bolus q 30 min ×2), then 0.5–5 mg/h (start 25% of loading dose/h). Onset (IV): 1–5 min, Peak (IM): 30–60 min, T ½ :1–4 h.	—
Phenobarbital	Phenobarbital 200 mg IV/SQ ×1 (or 10 mg/kg IV/SQ ×1), then 10–25 mg/h titrate up to 100 mg/h.	—
Propofol	20–50 mg × 1, then 10 mg/h and increase by 10 mg/h q 15 min as needed. (1 mcg/kg/min with 15 minute titration of 0.5 mcg/kg/min, may skip bolus).	Wears off within 10–30 minutes of discontinuation. Use large-bore IV due to pain at injection site.

GRIEF AND BEREAVEMENT

I. **Background information**
  A. Grief
    1. The emotional process of reacting to any type of loss
    2. Often the result of bereavement (the reality of being deprived from a loved one due to death), but can be due to other types of loss (such as a limb or a marriage)
    3. Mourning is the external display of grief
        a. Influenced by one's beliefs, religion, and cultural context
        b. The process one goes through adapting to the loss

4. Anticipatory (or preparatory) grief
   a. A normal type of grief reaction that occurs in anticipation of an impending loss, such as depression, heightened concern for the dying person (intensified attachment prior to the actual loss), rehearsal of the death, and completing unfinished business (forgiveness, goodbyes, expressions of love)
   b. Postdeath grief is not necessarily reduced with anticipatory grief, but unanticipated loss (i.e., anticipatory state not present) leads to a more complicated postdeath course (difficulty with accepting the loss, the world is without order, unable to grasp the full implications)
5. Uncomplicated (or normal) grief
   a. Immediately includes numbness, shock, disbelief, and/or denial.
   b. Marked by a gradual movement toward acceptance of the loss.
   c. Severe anxiety from the separation can occur resulting in dreams, illusions, anger, sadness, crying, despair, insomnia, anorexia, fatigue, guilt, and adjustments to daily routine (while daily functioning is very difficult, basic daily activities continue).
   d. Grief bursts (pangs) are 20–30-minute time-limited periods of intense distress.
      i. Can be unexpected or triggered by various reminders of the deceased person
   e. Over time common grief symptoms occur less frequently, become less intense, and are of briefer duration, typically anywhere from 6 months to 2 years after the loss.
6. Grief in children
   a. Children react to loss differently than adults, with grief often appearing for brief intermittent periods and marked more by behavior than words.

TABLE 7.10 Reactions to Loss by Age Group

Age Group	Behavior
Infants	Listlessness, quietness, weight loss, lack of sleep.
2–3 years	Confuse death with sleep, anxiety about sleeping. Loss of speech.
3–6 years	View death as a kind of sleep, worried about how the deceased are eating, toileting, breathing, or playing. Appetite, sleep, and bowel habits may change. Sometimes feel responsible ("Did I do something bad?"). Tantrums.
6–9 years	Increased curiosity about death, seen as final, however it happens to others. Increased learning problems, phobias, antisocial behaviors. Regressive behaviors.
9–12 years and older	No longer viewed as a punishment. Death seen as inevitable for all of us. Anxiety over own death, mood swings, sleeping problems, regressive behaviors.

II. Evaluation

A. Focuses on identifying risk factors for complicated grief
   1. Stages of grief have been proposed to help in the evaluation.
      a. Utility is limited as each patient and family have unique characteristics.
      b. Important to identify if depression is present.
         i. Depression has a more persistent flat affect, distorted self-esteem, overwhelming worthlessness, inability to shift hopes, and anhedonia (inability to feel pleasure).

TABLE 7.11 Grief Models

Kubler-Ross Model	Jacobs Stage Theory of Grief
Identifies stages, not a proposed sequence	Describes a proposed sequence
Denial – "I feel fine." "This can't be happening." **Anger** – "Why me?" "It's not fair!" **Bargaining** – "Just let me live to see my children graduate." **Depression** – "Why bother?" "I'm going to die, what's the point?" **Acceptance** – "I can't fight it, I may as well prepare for it."	Numbness-Disbelief Separation Distress (yearning, anger) Depression-Mourning Recovery

   2. Complicated grief has various types and definitions.
      a. Formal diagnostic criteria may be incorporated into *DSM-V* (pending publication May 2013).
      b. Red flags include denial for more than a few months, excessive drinking or drug use, antisocial behavior, suicidal threats, psychotic symptoms, acting as if the deceased is still here, and prolonged avoidance of potential triggers or reminders.
         i. Occurs in 15% of patients
      c. Risk factors
         i. Age <60 years
         ii. Limited social support or geographic separation from social supports
         iii. History of depression or other psychiatric illnesses
         iv. Lower income
         v. Pessimistic thinking
         vi. Insecure social attachment styles
         vii. Men (often due to limited social circles)
         viii. Women with young children at home
         ix. Anger
         x. Loss of a child
         xi. Unexpected death or loss
         xii. Financial stressors

B. Inhibited (absent or masked) grief is when there is little external evidence of a normal or expected grief response.
  - May be within the normal range of a response to loss, but can be masked by anxiety, depression, withdrawal, somatization, and avoidance
C. Delayed grief occurs at a much later time than expected.
  1. This may also be a normal human protective response to loss.
  2. Can occur months to years later.
D. Chronic grief or prolonged grief disorder is grief occurring for longer than 6 months, but typically lasting for more than 1–2 years.
E. Distorted (exaggerated) grief is characterized by extremely intense symptoms, often worsening with time (phobias, panic attacks, and irrational despair).

III. Management

TABLE 7.12 Managing Grief for Different Groups

Adults (target patients and families at highest risk)	Normalize the grieving process and validate emotional pain and grief. Facilitate normal grieving by being honest when discussing prognosis, goals, and treatment options. Listen and find out what or how much a patient or family wants to know, and once clarified, don't be ambiguous. Ask: "How are you doing with this news?" "Tell me what is going through your mind." Contact a social worker, chaplain, psychologist, or psychiatrist as appropriate for assistance and counseling services.
Children	Use simple, accurate terms like *death* and *died*. Avoid terms that can have dual meaning to an adult but easily be misunderstood by a child (e.g., "he is finally sleeping" or "passed away" or "we lost him" or "she's at rest"). Address feelings of guilt (children often feel responsible) and security (children need to feel safe and cared for). Children should be offered but not forced to take part in and plan for rituals. If the child wishes to participate in rituals, clearly explain what they will hear and see. If possible identify a close adult family member and/or friend to stay with the child during the ritual (such as a funeral). Be patient, allow for, be open to hear about, and inquire about emotions. Keep routines as stable as possible. Treat coexisting depression and anxiety medically as appropriate.

(continues)

TABLE 7.12 *(continued)*

Healthcare professionals	It is crucial to allow adequate personal time to grieve and heal as providers are often seeing their next patient before even having time to process their own emotions after events such as delivering bad news, acknowledging treatment failures, assisting suffering patients, and coping after their patient has died. Risk is highest amongst those sacrificing personal renewal time to meet the needs of patients. Regular meetings with colleagues to discuss grief, mistakes, suffering, and challenges can be rewarding. Eating healthy foods, exercising, pursuing hobbies, protecting personal relationships, lightheartedness/humor, slowing down for simple pleasures, journaling, and developing spiritual practices are important sources of renewal.

IV. **Writing a condolence card**
   A. Write in longhand.
   B. Offer a statement of condolence.
   C. Include a statement of what you observed the patient to be.
   D. Tell any personal story about the patient from your direct care.
   E. Include a statement of admiration, praise for care given by the family, or love they showed.
   F. Say something that you will always remember about your patient.

DEPRESSION

I. **Background information**
   A. Depression
      1. According to *DSM-IV*, having at least 5 out of 9 of the following symptoms for at least 2 weeks, including at least 1 of the first 2 criteria:
         a. Depressed mood
         b. Anhedonia (loss of interest)
         c. Weight change of >5% in 1 month
         d. Insomnia or hypersomnia
         e. Psychomotor agitation or retardation
         f. Fatigue
         g. Worthlessness or inappropriate guilt
         h. Poor concentration
         i. Suicidal ideation
      2. In palliative care the classic triad of hopelessness, helplessness, and worthlessness is helpful in differentiating depression from grief.
         a. Grief is due to a loss.
         b. Triad is often more helpful than somatic symptoms that are also commonly associated with a chronic illness (such as weight changes, fatigue, poor concentration, and sleep disturbances) or symptoms associated with medication side effects.

II. Evaluation

TABLE 7.13 Risk Factors for Depression

Pain	Personal or Family History	Alcoholism
Stroke (esp. left hemispheric)	Cancer (esp. pancreatic)	ESRD
Parkinson's disease	Diabetes	Heart attack
Multiple sclerosis	Hypothyroidism	Certain medications such as clonidine and beta-blockers

A. Interview
  1. Ask the following 2 screening questions:
     a. Are you depressed?
     b. Have you lost an interest in (or no longer enjoy) activities?
  2. If either is positive, take a more detailed history and keep a low threshold for initiating pharmacologic and/or nonpharmacologic interventions.

III. Management

A. Supportive psychotherapy
  1. Should be provided by anyone on the palliative care team with experience, including the physician, nurse, and/or social worker
  2. If appropriate, referrals to a chaplain, psychologist, or psychiatrist should be provided.
  3. Reinforcing nonabandonment and maximizing active listening is crucial.
  4. Encourage patients to talk about themselves and their lives and to feel free to ask questions and identify worries.
  5. Identify and mobilize the patient's own strengths and coping skills.
     a. Help the patient regain self-esteem, make peace with the past, and regain control of the situation as much as possible.

B. Pharmacotherapy

TABLE 7.14 Pharmacotherapy for Depression

Drug	Starting and Max. Dose	Comments
Psychostimulants		
Onset ranges from few hours up to 48 hours, can also stimulate appetite, can promote insomnia if given within 8 hours of bedtime, caution if heart disease or delirium, concomitant anxiety. Utilize if prognosis to weeks or if needed while SSRIs/SNRIs are initiated.		
Dextroamphetamine	10 mg PO q am and titrate weekly by 10 mg up to 60 mg PO q am.	—
Methylphenidate	5 mg (2.5 mg elderly) PO q am and titrate every other day up to 40 mg/day divide twice per day (2nd dose no later than noon).	First-line psychostimulant. Not much efficacy seen over 40 mg/day.
Modafinil	200 mg PO q am, max 300 mg PO q am.	Nonamphetamine mechanism. Consider only for cancer patients if methylphenidate contraindicated or has excessive side effects.

(continues)

TABLE 7.14 (*continued*)

Drug	Starting and Max. Dose	Comments
SSRIs Usually well tolerated, takes effect in 3–6 weeks, may decrease pain, most common side effect is GI distress and sexual dysfunction, must be titrated when discontinued.		
Citalopram	20 mg PO daily, max 40 mg daily.	Least drug-drug interactions. Increased risk for QTc prolongation, especially with doses >40 mg/day.
Escitalopram	10 mg PO daily, max 20 mg daily.	Least drug-drug interactions.
Fluoxetine	20 mg PO q am, max 60 mg q am.	Longest to steady state among the SSRIs. Can be activating. Avoid use with tamoxifen.
Paroxetine	10 mg PO q pm, max 60 mg PO q pm.	Can be sedating. High risk of withdrawal due to short T ½. Avoid use with tamoxifen.
Sertraline	25 mg PO q am, max 200 mg PO q am.	Can be activating.
SNRIs Activating, takes effect in 3–6 weeks, may decrease pain, most common side effect is GI distress.		
Duloxetine	20 mg PO daily, max 60 mg daily (can divide twice daily).	Doses >60 mg/day have not shown benefit. May be helpful also for neuropathies.
Venlafaxine	37.5 mg PO q am-twice daily, max 150 mg twice daily (extended release 37.5 mg PO q am, max 225 mg daily).	May reduce hot flashes in cancer patients. May be helpful for neuropathies. Can increase haloperidol concentrations.
Other		
Buproprion	100 mg PO twice daily, max 450 mg/day (SR: 150 mg PO daily, max 400 mg/day; XL: 150 mg PO q am, max 450 mg daily).	Lowers seizure threshold. May increase risk of weight loss. Activating. Avoid use with tamoxifen.
Mirtazapine	7.5 mg PO at bedtime, max 60 mg at bedtime.	Oral dissolving tab available. May be used to augment SSRI/SNRIs. Can improve appetite/weight gain/insomnia. Lower doses more sedating.
Trazodone	25 mg PO q pm, max 600 mg PO at bedtime (divide higher doses three times daily).	Sedating. Risk for orthostatic hypotension and priapism.

(continues)

TABLE 7.14 (*continued*)

Drug	Starting and Max. Dose	Comments
Other (*continued*)		
Buspirone	2.5 mg PO twice daily and titrate up to 60 mg daily.	Augmentation of other interventions.
Lithium	Start 300 mg PO twice daily and titrate up to 900 mg/day (goal blood level of 0.6–1 meq/L).	Consider only for patients with prognosis measured in years due to multiple drug interactions and need for routine monitoring. Use for augmentation of other interventions. Baseline and q 6 months TSH, CBC, Bun/Creatinine, lytes. Baseline ECG age >50 (or history of cardiac problems). Weekly lithium levels (12 hours post dose) until stable for 2 weeks, then monthly for 6 months, then quarterly.
Triiodothyronine	25–50 mcg/day.	Augmentation of other interventions.
Ketamine	0.5 mg/kg IV single dose.	Consider for refractory depression. Can see response within 1–2 hours and last up to a week. Consult experienced provider prior to use.
TCAs		
Generally avoid in elderly, takes effect in 3–6 weeks; all have significant drug-drug interactions, if needed desipramine and nortriptyline are best tolerated as least anticholinergic; drug levels can be obtained and monitor EKGs as appropriate; common side effects include anticholinergic effects, sedation, orthostatic hypotension/falls, arrhythmias, and weight gain.		
Amitriptyline	10 mg PO at bedtime, max 300 PO at bedtime.	–
Desipramine	10 mg PO at bedtime, max 300 mg PO at bedtime.	Less risk of side effects compared to imipramine.
Doxepin	10 mg PO at bedtime, max 300 mg PO at bedtime.	–
Imipramine	25 mg PO at bedtime, max 300 mg PO at bedtime.	–
Nortriptyline	10 mg PO at bedtime, max 150 mg PO at bedtime.	Less risk of side effects compared to amitriptyline.

B. Psychiatry referral triggers
- Uncertainty as to diagnosis, history of or underlying major psychiatric disorder, suicidal, psychotic, delirious, or unresponsive to therapy

FATIGUE

I. Background information
A. Fatigue (asthenia)
- An unusual persistent subjective sense of tiredness despite adequate rest that interferes with usual functioning
  a. Associated with the inability to initiate, decreased concentration, and increased emotional lability
  b. Strongly associated with cachexia, malnutrition, and lean muscle mass loss

II. Evaluation
A. Obtain a thorough history and explore descriptions of fatigue (tired, loss of energy, exhaustion) and impact on function
1. Have patient rate fatigue on a scale of 1–10 and treat if ≥4.
2. Identify possible etiologies such as anemia, electrolyte abnormalities, chronic hypoxia, nutritional deficiencies, infection, myopathies, endocrinopathies (such as hypothyroidism and hypogonadism), depression, sleep disturbances, and medication side effects.
3. Document patient-reported 0–10 scale and the ECOG performance scale for cancer patients.

III. Management
A. Nonpharmacologic methods
1. Establish achievable goals of daily living, obtain assistive medical equipment (wheelchair, walker, hospital bed, bedside commode), and physical and occupational therapy as tolerated (also for learning energy conservation techniques).
2. Increase exposure to sunlight if tolerated and fresh air, and encourage maintenance and range-of-motion exercise (which is the only proven therapy). Recent reports that a broader range of exercise improves quality of life scores thus increased physical activity should be encouraged as tolerated.
3. Treat identified etiologies considering underlying disease process and if consistent with patient's goals of care (such as erythropoietin for anemia).

TABLE 7.15 Pharmacologic Interventions for Fatigue

Drug	Dose	Comments
Dexamethasone	4–8 mg PO q am 2 weeks.	Effect should last up to 4 weeks after completion. Use if prognosis measured in months. Keep in mind small risk of steroid-induced myopathy especially if used > a few months. Due to long T ½ dosing can be qam to minimize insomnia.
Prednisone	40 mg PO daily for 2 weeks.	Use if prognosis measured in months.
Megace	160–800 mg PO daily.	Caution due to increased venous thromboembolism risk. Use for patients with prognosis > a few months.
Methylphenidate	2.5–5 mg PO q am and 2.5–5 mg PO q noon, max 40 mg/day.	Can be dosed 5 mg PO q 2 h, up to 4 ×/day. Useful for opioid-induced fatigue; unclear if beneficial for cancer-related fatigue.
Dexmethylphenidate (d-isomer of methylphenidate)	See methylphenidate dosing.	—
Dextroamphetamine	2.5 mg PO daily up to 20 mg/day.	Can consider using as needed a few hours before an event (such as a wedding).
Modafinil (Provigil)	100 mg po q am and titrate up to 400 mg/ day PO.	Use for shift work sleep disorder, sleep apnea, and narcolepsy. Can also be tried for multiple sclerosis–, HIV-, ALS-related fatigue, and cancer patients with severe fatigue. Second-line agent to methylphenidate. Studies show most consistent benefit only with cancer patients.
Midodrine	10 PO three times per day.	For treating autonomic failure with postural hypotension.
Fish oils (omega-3 fatty acids)	500–3000 mg/day.	For potential anticytokine activity. Caution if low blood pressure (may lower).
Testosterone	Dosing varies based on testosterone level and dosage form used.	Commonly low in men with cancer, have low threshold for measuring and treating if low. Contraindicated in prostate cancer.
Donepezil	5 mg PO q am.	Consider for opioid-induced sedation.
Thalidomide	100 mg po 4 ×/day.	Used for advanced HIV patients with concurrent cachexia and for anticytokine activity. Prescribing restricted through REMS program.

INSOMNIA

I. **Background information**
   A. Quantitative or qualitative decrease in restorative sleep

II. **Evaluation**
   A. History of sleep stages involved, sleep hygiene, recent stressors, changes in medical or psychiatric conditions, and associated symptoms.
   B. Consider polysomnography if sleep apnea suspected.
   C. Evaluate for anxiety and/or depression.

III. **Management**
   A. Nonpharmacologic interventions
   - Progressive muscle relaxation therapy, using the bed only for sleep (no watching television or reading in bed), avoiding caffeine and other stimulants after lunch, avoiding alcohol and smoking in the evening, and try cognitive behavioral therapy
   B. Medication

TABLE 7.16 Pharmacologic Therapy for Insomnia

Drug	Dose	Comments
Benzodiazepines. Caution paradoxical agitation risk (especially elderly), amnesia, and rebound insomnia. Half-life 10–15 hours.		
Estazolam	0.5–2 mg PO at bedtime.	–
Flurazepam	15–30 mg PO at bedtime.	–
Lorazepam	2–4 mg PO at bedtime.	–
Temazepam	7.5–15 mg PO at bedtime.	–
Triazolam	0.125–0.25 mg PO at bedtime.	–
Non-benzodiazepine hypnotics		
Eszopiclone	2–3 mg PO at bedtime.	For sleep onset insomnia, use 3 mg dose for sleep maintenance insomnia. Decrease dose for 3A4 inhibitors.
Zaleplon	5–20 mg PO at bedtime (max 10 mg in elderly).	For sleep onset insomnia.
Zolpidem	10 mg PO at bedtime (5 mg in elderly). Extended-release: 12.5 mg PO at bedtime (6.25 mg in elderly).	For sleep onset insomnia. Use extended-release formulation for sleep maintenance insomnia.

(continues)

TABLE 7.16 (*continued*)

Drug	Dose	Comments
Antidepressants		
Doxepin	10–50 mg PO at bedtime.	–
Imipramine	10–75 mg PO at bedtime.	–
Mirtazapine	7.5–15 mg PO at bedtime.	–
Trazadone	25–100 mg PO at bedtime.	–
Antihistamines		
Diphenhydramine	25–100 mg PO at bedtime.	Avoid in elderly
Other		
Melatonin	Start 0.3 mg PO at bedtime, double dose weekly, max 10 mg.	For sleep efficiency (age-related insomnia). Avoid in dementia patients, seizure disorder, children, or in those taking anticoagulants.
Ramelteon	8 mg PO at bedtime.	Melatonin agonist. Caution if hepatic impairment. Consider for chronic, severe sleep-onset difficulty in patients with good prognosis (>few months) and not due to reversible etiologies.
Pramipexole	0.125 mg PO 1 h prior to bedtime. Max 0.5 mg.	For restless leg syndrome can also consider ropinirole 0.25–4 mg/day or levodopa/carbidopa 25/100. Adjunctive agents for restless leg syndrome include clonazepam 0.5 mg and iron supplementation (even if not iron deficient).

DEFINITIONS

I. **Background information**
   A. Pain is the unpleasant sensory and emotional experience with actual or potential damage or described in terms of such damage.
      - It is subjective, being whatever the person says it is, existing whenever the person says it does.
   B. Total pain (suffering) consists of 4 components, each of which can contribute to a patient's perception and tolerance of pain. The mnemonic PAIN is helpful to remember each component:
      P: Physical pain (results in loss of bodily control)
      A: Anxiety (psychiatric/emotional component), depression
      I: Interpersonal (social component), guilt, loss of trust, stressors (family, friends, work, financial, and self-worth)
      N: Not accepting (spiritual component), existential distress, hope, meaning

PAIN DESCRIPTORS

I. **Nociceptive pain (somatic or visceral)**
   A. Generated by a noxious stimulus (thermal, mechanical, or chemical) and sensed by a nerve fiber.
   B. Somatic pain is localized and due to soft tissue damage, such as originating from muscle, skin, and bone.
      1. Superficial somatic pain is sharp and prick-like.
      2. Deep somatic pain is aching, stabbing, and throbbing.
   C. Visceral pain is poorly localized, frequently radiates, and is due to stretch, inflammation, or ischemia of internal organs resulting in deep, dull, gnawing, squeezing, cramp-like pain.
      - Examples include peptic ulcer disease, biliary colic, angina, appendicitis, pleurisy, and urinary retention.
   D. Nociceptive pain can be described as being due to inflammatory, mechanical/compressive, or musculoskeletal etiologies.
   E. Nociceptive signals travel to the dorsal horn of the spinal cord, then ascend via the spinothalamic tract to the thalamus then on to the cortex, amygdala, and cerebellum.
II. **Neuropathic pain**
   A. Pain that results from direct injury to a nerve fiber.
   B. Central nervous system etiologies include post-stroke pain and phantom limb pain.

C. Peripheral nerve etiologies include various neuropathies and postherpetic neuralgia (i.e., poly- and mononeuropathies).
D. Neuropathic pain associated with autonomic changes is considered complex regional pain.
   1. Described as burning, electric shocks, shooting pain.
   2. On exam may find allodynia (pain from nonpainful stimuli), hyperalgesia (increased perception of painful stimuli), or other neurological findings.

ASSESSMENT

I. Summary mnemonic "ABC"
   A. **A**sk (take history using the 4 As):
      1. Analgesia (pain history).
      2. ADLs (impact on life).
      3. Adverse effects (of interventions).
      4. Aberrant behavior (addiction risk).
   B. **B**elieve the patient's history.
   C. **C**hoose medication or intervention to try.
II. Words to Use
   A. Avoid using terms like *pain sufferer* or *pain patient, narcotics, drugs,* and *painkillers.*
   B. Instead, use terms such as *people living with pain* or *person with pain, opioids, medicines,* and *pain relievers or analgesics.*
      1. "Tell me about your pain/aches/soreness/discomfort."
      2. "Tell me how you take your pain medicines."
      3. "Can you describe your pain? How does it feel?"

DOCUMENTING PAIN

I. Adults
   A. Utilize a 0–10 visual analog pain scale.
      • "What does your pain feel like?" Utilize a 0–10 scale on a thermometer or ruler for example or a numerical rating scale: "On a scale of 0–10, with 10 being worst possible pain."
   B. For nonverbal adults, such as patients with dementia: Utilize a nonverbal scale that assesses breathing patterns, vocalizations, facial expression, body language, and consolability to determine severity of pain.
II. Children
   A. For infants or nonverbal children: Similar to nonverbal adults utilize a nonverbal (i.e., observational) scale.
   B. For children ages 3–8: Utilize a facial image-based scale.
   C. For children 8–11: Utilize a visual-analog 0–10 scale.

D. For adolescents: Utilize adult scales.
   1. Describe and document the pain.
   2. Useful mnemonics include "OLD CARTS" or "PQRSTU":
      a. **O**nset, **L**ocation, **D**uration, **C**haracter, **A**lleviating/**A**ggravating factors, **R**adiating, **T**emporal factors, **S**everity.
      b. **P**alliative/**P**recipitating factors, **Q**uality, **R**adiation, **S**everity, **T**emporal pattern, "**U**" You /impact on life.

III. Breakthrough pain
A. 3 types
   1. Incident pain: Anticipate and premedicate.
   2. Idiopathic: Add an around-the-clock adjuvant and/or non-opioid analgesic.
   3. End-of-dose failure: Increase frequency of long-acting agent.

MANAGEMENT OF PAIN

I. 3 Steps
A. Assess all types of pain (total pain).
B. Treat all types of pain.
C. Frequent reassessment.

II. WHO Ladder
A. This is not a ladder to climb, but rather where to start based on initial pain intensity.
B. Adjuvants can be utilized as needed at any step.
C. Step 1: Mild pain (rated 1–3)
   • Start with acetaminophen or NSAIDs.
D. Step 2: Moderate pain (rated 4–7)
   1. Start with weak opioids such as tramadol or codeine.
   2. Consider combination opioid products (with hydrocodone, oxycodone, or codeine).
E. Step 3: Severe pain (rated 8–10)
   • Start with strong opioids such as morphine, oxycodone, hydromorphone, fentanyl, or methadone.

NSAIDS AND ACETAMINOPHEN

I. NSAID comments
A. Side effects include inhibiting platelet aggregation (caution if CAD or high thrombotic risk), dyspepsia gastric ulceration, nephrotoxicity (use with caution if chronic kidney disease, hypertension, or heart failure present), liver toxicity, and allergic reactions.
B. GI toxicity can be minimized with misoprostol, H2 blockers, and proton pump inhibitors, in those with risk factors or on high-dose NSAIDs.

    C. Consider avoiding NSAIDs if >2 of these risk factors
        1. History of ulceration.
        2. Age >60 years.
        3. Taking concurrent glucocorticoids.
        4. Taking anticoagulants or aspirin.

TABLE 8.1 Non-Opioid Analgesics

Drug	Dosing	Comments
Acetaminophen	Infants: (Max 75 mg/kg daily) PO/PR 10–15 mg/kg/dose q 6 h IV (not studied in infants): suggested 33% reduction and if <1 month old 50% reduction from children's dose (7.5–15 mg/kg/dose q 6 h (Max: 60 mg/kg/day)	For adult IV dosing pain relief is approximate to 30 mg ketorolac or morphine 0.1 mg/kg
	Children (ages 2–12 or adults <50 kg): (Max 2600 mg daily) PO/PR: 10–15 mg/kg/dose q 6 h IV: 15 mg/kg q 6 h or 12.5 mg/kg q 4 h (max 3,750 mg/day if <50 kg)	
	Adults (≥50 kg): Max: 4000 mg/day (2000 mg if liver disease) PO/PR: 325–1000 mg q 6 h IV: 1000 mg q 6 h or 650 mg q 4 h. (ESRD dose q 8–12 h)	
NSAIDs—Carboxylic Acids		
Acetylsalicylic acid (aspirin)	Children: 10–15 mg/kg PO/PR q 4–6 h (Max 4 g/day) Adults: PO 325–650 mg q 4–6 h (Max 4 g/day) PR 300–600 mg q 4–6 h (Max 4 g/day)	–
Salsalate	Adults: 500–750 mg PO q 8–12 h (Max 3 g/day)	Lower GI risk profile; does not interfere with platelet aggregation
Choline magnesium trisalicylate	Children (<37 kg): 25 mg/kg PO q 12 h Adults: 500–1500 mg PO q 8–12 h, or 3 g PO at bedtime	Lower GI risk profile; does not interfere with platelet aggregation

(continues)

TABLE 8.1 (*continued*)

Drug	Dosing	Comments
NSAIDs—Propionic Acids		
Ibuprofen	Infants >6 months/children: 4–10 mg/kg PO q 6–8 h (Max 40 mg/kg/day) Adults PO: 200–400 mg q 4–6 h (Max 2.4 g/day) IV (Caldolor): 400–800 q 6 h (Max 3.2 g; ensure well hydrated)	–
Ketoprofen	Adults PO: 50 mg q 6 h or 75 mg q 8 h or 200 mg ER daily (Max 300 mg/day)	–
Naproxen	Children 2–12 years old: 5 mg/kg PO q 12 h Adults: 500 mg PO ×1, then 250 mg PO q 6 h (Max 1250 mg/day)	–
NSAIDs—Acetic Acids		
Indomethacin	Children ≥2 years: 1–2 mg/kg/day PO in 2–4 divided doses (Max 4 mg/kg/day up to 150–200 mg/day) Adults: 25–50 mg PO q 8–12 h (Max 200 mg/day)	–
Sulindac	Adults: 150 mg–200 mg PO q 12 h	–
Diclofenac	PO: capsule 25 mg q 6 h or tablet 50 mg q 8 h 1% Topical gel: 4 g to lower extremities q 6 h, 2 g to upper extremities (Max total body dose 32 g/day) Patch: 1 patch q 12 h to area of maximum acute pain	–
Etodolac	Children: 0–30 kg: 400 mg ER PO daily 1–45 kg: 600 mg ER PO daily 46–60 kg: 800 mg ER PO daily Adults: 200–400 mg PO q 6–8 h (Max 1000 mg/day)	For children with juvenile idiopathic arthritis usually see response within 2 weeks
Ketorolac (Toradol)	Adults, PO: (transitioning from IV formulation) 20 mg PO ×1, then 10 mg q 4–6 h as needed (Max 40 mg/day; use 10 mg loading dose if age >65 or if weight <50 kg) IV/IM 30 mg q 6 h up to 5 days (use 15 mg if age >65 or if weight <50 kg)	–

(*continues*)

TABLE 8.1 (*continued*)

Drug	Dosing	Comments
NSAIDs-Fenamates		
Meclofenamate	50 mg PO q 4–6 h (Max 400 mg/day)	May take 2–3 weeks to see max benefit
NSAIDs-Oxicams (enolic acids)		
Meloxicam (partial Cox-2)	Children (≥2 yrs, juvenile idiopathic arthritis): 0.125 mg/kg PO daily (Max 7.5 mg/day) Adults: 7.5–15 mg PO daily	–
Piroxicam	Children 0.2–0.3 mg/kg PO daily (Max 15 mg/day) Adults: 10–20 mg PO daily or divided twice per day (Max 20 mg/day)	–
NSAIDs-Naphylkanones		
Nabumetone	Adults 500–1000 mg PO q 12–24 h (Max 2000 mg/day)	Lower GI risk profile
NSAIDs-Cox-2 inhibitors		
Celecoxib	Children 10–25 kg: 50 mg PO q 12 h, >25 kg: 100 mg PO q 12 h Adults: Loading 400 mg PO ×1, with optional 200 mg in 12 h if needed on day 1. Maintenance 100–200 mg PO q 12 h (can skip loading dose)	Does not interfere with platelet aggregation

OPIOIDS

I. Prescribing tips
   A. Acute mild to moderate pain or chronic mild pain: Utilize prn (as needed) dosing regimens
   B. Acute severe pain or chronic moderate to severe pain: Utilize a basal regimen (if under close observation) plus a prn dose equal to 5–15% of the 24-hour daily dose (for oral opioids)
   C. For opioid-naïve patients with acute pain crisis (under close observation)
      1. PO: Morphine IR 5 mg, hydromorphone 1 mg, or oxycodone 5 mg q 1 h until pain controlled.
      2. IV: Morphine 1 mg, hydromorphone 0.2 mg, or fentanyl 20 mcg q 1 minute up to 10 minutes, then wait 5 minutes before repeating cycle until acute pain crisis controlled.
         a. If after 30 doses pain still not controlled, if resp. rate <10 breaths/minute, or if becoming sedated, continue investigation into etiology of acute pain crisis.
         b. If utilizing SQ for acute pain crisis, use IV dosing with 5-minute spacing with same precautions.

3. Pain is controlled when pain score drops 2–4 points from initial score (not until pain is completely relieved).

D. Titration due to escalating chronic pain

1. Breakthrough dosing baseline should be 5–15% (usually 10%) of the 24-h total opioid routine dosing utilizing a short-acting agent.

2. For ongoing pain (e.g., if after a third breakthrough dose pain continues), increase the breakthrough dose by 25–50% (mild–moderate pain) or 50–100% (moderate–severe pain).

   a. Once pain is controlled, calculate the new 24-hour daily dose for the long-acting agent (scheduled + breakthrough doses = new daily scheduled dose, but no greater than 100%; change every 24 h and no more frequent than every 72 h for fentanyl patch, methadone, and levorphanol).

   b. If adverse effects develop, switch to a new opioid.

      i. If pain controlled, reduce new opioid by 25–50% of equianalgesic dose.

      ii. If pain is severe, utilize calculated equianalgesic dose for new opioid without adjusting for incomplete cross-tolerance.

E. Remember the bowels and utilize a stimulant laxative

F. Patient-controlled analgesia (PCA): IV or SQ

1. Include hourly basal rate, if appropriate (i.e., opioid-tolerant for >7 days or anticipated chronic need such as with cancer patients).

   a. Caution if opioid-naïve, elderly, morbidly obese, postop or sleep apnea risk.

   b. If needed, consider continuous O_2 monitoring depending on risk and goals of care.

   c. Include a loading dose when initiating or increasing a basal rate.

   d. Basal rates should be adjusted no more then every 8 hours (allow time to reach steady state between each change of basal rate).

2. Demand or bolus dose should be 50–150% of basal rate.

   a. Demand dose can be titrated every 30–60 minutes until desired effect is achieved (with acceptable toxicities).

3. Lockout/dosing interval (most will do well with 10 minutes).

4. For actively dying patients, allow family or nursing staff to administer for uncontrolled symptoms or prior to bathing/turning.

5. Adjust/titrate basal rate no more than every 8 hours, (i.e., time to steady state) and no more than a 100% change.

6. SQ tissue can absorb up to 3mL/h: Utilize a 25–27-gauge butterfly needle (upper arm, shoulder, abdomen, or thigh) up to a week at a time if tolerating.

[SEE OPIOID EQUIANALGESIC TABLE—Pages 162–163]

II. **Morphine**
  A. Neonates
    • IV 0.05 mg/kg q 4–8 h, max 0.1 mg/kg/dose. Infuse at 0.01 mg/kg/hour (10 mcg/kg/hour), max 0.02 mg/kg/hour.
  B. Infants/Children (>3 months)
    1. PO 0.2–0.5 mg/kg q 4–6 h.
    2. IV 0.1 mg/kg IV q 2 h or Infusion at 0.03 mg/kg/hour (30 mcg/kg/hour). Max: infants 2 mg/dose, 1–6 years 4 mg/dose, 7–12 years 8 mg/dose, adolescents 15 mg/dose.
  C. Adults
    1. Starting dose PO/SL 5–30 mg q 3 h (note: SL slower onset than PO, indicating largely swallowed/poor mucosal absorption/delayed liver activation of active metabolites).
    2. Once-daily PO (ideal for patients unable to swallow standard morphine formulations): Kadian (delayed onset) or Avinza (rapid-onset).
      a. Both capsules can be opened and granules can be sprinkled on applesauce (do not chew, crush, or dissolve granules).
      b. Kadian can be suspended in water and delivered via gastrostomy tube (size ≥16 F).

III. **Hydromorphone**
  A. Infants (>6 months and >10 kg).
    1. PO 0.03–0.06 mg/kg q 4 h.
    2. IV 0.01 mg/kg/dose q 3 h, infuse at 0.003–0.005 mg/kg/hour.
  B. Children/adolescents (<50 kg)
    1. PO 0.03–0.08 mg/kg q 3 h.
    2. IV 0.015 mg/kg q 3 h, infusion at 0.003–0.005 mg/kg/hour. (Max 0.2 mg/hour).
  C. Adults
    1. PO starting dose: 2–4 mg q 3 h.
    2. IV starting dose: 0.2–0.6 mg q 2 h, infusion usual dose 0.5–1 mg/h (or 7–15 mcg/kg/hour).

IV. **Levorphanol (also an NMDA antagonist and monoamine reuptake inhibitor)**
  A. Half-life is approximately 11 hours reaching steady state in about 3 days.
  B. Peaks in 30 minutes after IV dosing or 1 hour after oral dosing, no reported QT prolongation, can be crushed and given via G-tube.
  C. Adults: 6 mg PO total daily dose if opioid-naïve (dividing dose q 6–12 h depending on length of pain relief).

D. Ratio of morphine to levorphanol to use varies depending on volume of 24-hour oral morphine
   1. Less than 100 mg, 12:1
   2. 100–299 mg, 15:1
   3. 300–599 mg, 20:1
   4. 600–799 mg, 25:1
   5. Greater than 800mg, not studied

V. Oxycodone
A. Children (>6 months): 0.1–0.2 mg/kg PO q 3 h.
B. Adults.
   - Opioid-naïve: Controlled-release 10 mg PO q 12 h, titrate q 2 days.

VI. Oxymorphone
A. Adults: IR dosed q 6 h, ER dosed q 12 h.

VII. Fentanyl
A. Risk evaluation and mitigation strategy (REMS) required for all prescribers of transmucosal fentanyl products (access at www.tirfremsaccess.com to complete the process).
B. Oral transmucosal stick lozenge (Actiq): No conversion from fentanyl patch or IV.
   1. For breakthrough pain in opioid-tolerant patients on at least 60 mg oral morphine/day equivalent or 25-mcg/h patch. Place next to buccal mucosa between cheek and gum, move gently side to side if needed, and allow to dissolve, then remove handle (may remove lozenge earlier if adequate response noted or side effects noted).
   2. Peaks in 20–40 minutes and lasts 2–3 hours.
   3. 200-mcg dose ×1, then repeat if needed in 15 minutes (30 minutes after start of first dose).
      a. If two doses required, next breakthrough pain dose should be doubled (e.g., 400 mcg).
   4. Studied up to 4 doses/day; if more needed adjust basal opioid.
C. Oral buccal tablet (Fentora): No conversion from fentanyl patch or IV
   1. For breakthrough pain in opioid-tolerant patients on at least 60 mg oral morphine/day equivalent or 25-mcg/h patch.
   2. Place tablet between upper cheek and gum near rear molar. Should dissolve in 14–25 minutes, remnants may be swallowed with water. Do not chew, suck, break, or swallow tablets.
   3. Converting from transmucosal lozenges (Actiq)
      a. 200–400 mcg = 100 mcg Fentora
      b. 600–800 mcg = 200 mcg Fentora
      c. 1200–1600 mcg = 200 mcg ×2 Fentora (1 each side of mouth)

    4. Dosing: 100-mcg dose ×1, repeat 100-mcg dose in 30 minutes if needed. Wait 4 hours prior to third dose if needed (and can try next higher dose). Once above 400-mcg dose, titrate in 200-mcg increments.

D. Oral buccal film (Onsolis)

    1. No conversion, start 200 mcg ×1, repeat no more than q 2 hours and titrate up to 4 films (800 mcg).

    2. If more required, use 1200-mcg film for next episode.

    3. Can use up to 4 applications/day.

    4. Wet inside of cheek first (using tongue or water) and place pink side against moistened cheek using finger to hold in place for 5 seconds. Should dissolve within 15–30 minutes. Okay to drink liquids 5 minutes after application.

        a. If more than 1 film used simultaneously, apply 1 to each side of mouth. Do not cut, tear, chew, or swallow the film.

E. Nasal spray (Lazanda)

    1. No conversion, start all patients with 100 mcg dose in one nostril.

    2. If no relief in 30 minutes, then 2 hours after initial dose double the dose (e.g., 100 mcg per nostril = 200 mcg total).

    3. If no relief, double again in 2 hours to 400-mcg spray (studied up to 800-mcg dose).

    4. Once working dose identified, use that dose for subsequent exacerbations; limit to 4 doses/day.

    5. Prime spray into provided pouch (4 sprays with green bar showing when ready). Insert 1 cm into nostril and point toward bridge of nose (close off other nostril using 1 finger). Press until click is heard and counter advances by one (may not feel the spray). Do not blow nose for 30 minutes. Bottles have 8 sprays and should be disposed of appropriately if >5 days since last use (or 4 days after primed).

F. Sublingual tablet (Abstral)

    1. No conversion, start all patients with 100-mcg dose, repeat in 30 minutes if pain unrelieved.

    2. Wait 2 hours before treating another episode.

    3. Titrate in 100-mcg increments as needed up to 400 mcg, then in increments of 200 mcg (e.g., 400 mcg, then 600 mcg).

    4. Do not use more than 4 tablets any one time (studied up to 800 mcg); limit treatment to 4 episodes/day.

    5. Allow to completely dissolve; do not chew, suck, or swallow; do not eat or drink until completely dissolved.

        a. If mouth is dry, moisten mucosa with water just prior to administration sublingually.

G. Fentanyl transdermal patch (chronic pain)
1. Consider using patch in advanced renal failure patients, those unable to tolerate oral medications or other opioids, and for convenience and increasing compliance.
2. If titrating, no patch change should exceed 50 mcg/h; titrate after patch has reached steady state (q 2–3 days).
3. Some patients may require q 48 h dosing instead of q 72 h dosing.
4. Do not use for managing acute pain.
5. When discontinued takes approximately 17 h for 50% decrease in levels.
6. Calculating patch dose: 2 mg oral morphine/24 h = 1 mcg/h of transdermal patch (i.e., 50 mg oral morphine in 24 h = 25 mcg/h fentanyl patch).
7. Avoid patch unless on chronic opioids at an equianalgesic dose. Avoid initiating or titrating during acute pain exacerbations, fever, or cachexia (theoretical erratic absorption with severe cachexia due to fentanyl patch requires a subcutaneous fat store).
8. Apply patch to nonirritated skin with ample subcutaneous fat (chest, back, flank, upper arm). Avoid external heat sources near patch. May be covered with adhesive film if needed. Do not shave hair; use clippers if needed.

H. Fentanyl IV
1. Dosing is equivalent to patch dosing (25-mcg/h patch = 25-mcg/h IV infusion) however conversion is different (see Opioid Equianalgesic & Pharmacokinetic Table).
2. Children: 0.5–2 mcg/kg/dose q 1–2 h or infuse at 0.5–2 mcg/kg/hour and titrate as needed.
3. Adults:
   a. Acute pain flares can utilize 50–100 mcg IV demand doses q 6–15 min until pain controlled.
   b. Infusion start at 0.5–1.5 mcg/kg/hour (e.g., 25–200 mcg/h).
   c. PCA, start basal at ≤50 mcg/hour, demand 10–50 mcg, with lockout 6–8 min.
   d. Critically ill patients 0.7–10 mcg/kg/h (i.e., up to 700 mcg/hour if 70-kg patient) or 0.35–1.5 mcg/kg q 30 min (more frequent if ventilated).
4. From patch switching to fentanyl IV, remove patch from body and provide 50% IV bolus doses as needed for adequate breakthrough pain relief during first 6 hours, then start IV infusion at 50% of patch rate; 12 hours after patch removed can increase to original patch rate.
5. Switching to patch from IV fentanyl: Place patch on skin, then 6 hours later decrease IV infusion by 50%, then 12 hours after patch placed discontinue IV infusion.

VIII. Methadone

A. Also NMDA antagonist, inhibits norepinephrine and serotonin reuptake similar to some antidepressants, potential for relieving neuropathic pain as well.

B. Caution due to observed higher rate of respiratory depression (monitor closely due to long half-life up to 190 hours).

C. Caution due to cardiac conduction abnormalities (due to prolonged QTc).

D. Indications: Pain refractory to other opioids, intractable side effects with other opioids (such as true morphine allergies), untenable costs of other opioids, advanced renal failure, and possible added relief of neuropathic or hyperalgesia-related pain.

E. Relative contraindications (some depend on goals of care): Limited prognosis measured in days; lives alone; unreliable historian; history of noncompliance, syncope, cardiac arrhythmias, or structural heart disease.

F. EKG recommendations: Baseline screening EKG, follow-up in 30 days then annually (or when titrating above 100 mg/day or if unexplained syncope or seizure-like symptoms). If QTc 450–500 ms, discuss and document risks/benefits with patient and monitor more frequently; if >500 ms consider discontinuing or reducing dose, ensure normokalemic.

G. Metabolized by cP450 system, examples (not inclusive) of effect on methadone level include:

1. Increased levels (i.e., reduce dose by ≥25% and encourage rescue medication usage): fluconazole, ketoconazole, amiodarone, erythromycin, clarithromycin, diltiazem, verapamil, citalopram, paroxetine, fluoxetine, ciprofloxacin, amitriptyline

2. Decreased levels (keep current dose but encourage rescue medication usage): barbiturates, carbamazepine, nevirapine, phenytoin, rifampin, spironolactone

H. Dosing:

1. Children (>6 months): 0.1 mg/kg PO/IV q 6 h

2. Opioid-naïve adults

   a. Conservative approach: 2.5–5 mg PO q 8–12 h, titrate by 50% q 4–7 days; utilize an alternative short-acting opioid for breakthrough pain.

   b. Loading dose approach: 5–10 mg PO q 4 h prn only. On day 8, calculate the prior 24-h usage and use that as your starting total daily dosage. Ongoing prn dose then would be 10% of the daily dose q 1 h (max 5 breakthrough doses/day).

3. Converting to oral methadone: Calculate 24-h total oral morphine equivalent dose and divide by ratio ranging from 3–20 for total 24-h methadone dose. For additional safety margin can decrease result by 50–75% (multiply by 0.5 or 0.25, respectively)
   a. Stepwise method (monitor closely): Day 1, replace $1/3$ of current opioid with $1/3$ methadone dose; day 2, replace another $1/3$ with another $1/3$ of methadone; day 3, complete conversion to methadone.
   b. Ratio of morphine to methadone to use varies depending on volume of 24-hour oral morphine
      i. Less than 101 mg, 3:1
      ii. 101–300 mg, 5:1
      iii. 301–600 mg, 10:1
      iv. 601–800 mg, 12:1
      v. 801–1000 mg, 15:1
      vi. Greater than 1000 mg, 20:1
4. Converting FROM oral methadone TO oral morphine: 3:1 oral morphine:methadone is consensus opinion (e.g., 15-mg daily dose methadone = 45-mg oral morphine/day). Start immediate-release morphine 12 hours after last methadone dose q 4 h with prn dose available q 2 h. In 4–7 days, should be able to calculate new basal dose of morphine for initiating a long-acting formulation.
5. Converting to IV methadone (i.e., PCA): Calculate 24-h oral methadone dose based on current opioid 24-h oral morphine equivalent usage, then divide 24-h oral methadone dose by 2 (2:1 ratio) for the 24-h IV methadone dose. This can be divided by 24 for the hourly infusion rate via PCA (preferred method versus q 6–8 h dosing). PCA demand dose would be the hourly rate given q 20–30 min. Backup clinician dose for breakthrough pain would be double the hourly rate. Basal rate should only be changed 12 hours after initiation or dose increases as analgesia/sedation can still be increasing.
   a. Suggested IV starting dose examples if already on IV infusion: Morphine 10 mg/h = methadone 1 mg/h; hydromorphone 1.5 mg/h = methadone 0.3 mg/h; fentanyl 250 mcg/h = methadone 1.25 mg/h.
   b. Use preservative-free IV methadone solution (if an available option) only for patients at highest risk of QT prolongation (unexplained syncope, seizures, congenital deafness, abnormal electrolytes, renal failure, cardiovascular disease, bradycardia, advanced age, female, heart failure, hypotension, myocardial ischemia, hypothermia, on known medications that will increase methadone levels, and pituitary insufficiency).

    c. For IV methadone get baseline EKG, then in 24 h, then at 4 days of initiation, dose increases, heart failure exacerbation, or new medications that may affect the QTc. Keep electrolytes normal. If QTc prolongation is noted, check for hypokalemia, hypomagnesemia, other contributing drugs, and for myocardial ischemia.

    d. Converting from IV methadone: Most likely oral:parenteral methadone ratio is 1:0.7. Calculate the 24-h dose of IV methadone and multiply by 1.3 to determine the 24-h dose of oral methadone. Give first dose of oral methadone at the time the IV methadone infusion is discontinued.

IX. Tramadol (has a ceiling effect and lowers the seizure threshold)

  A. Children (>6 months): 1–2 mg/kg PO q 4 h (max 400 mg/day)

  B. Adults with end-stage renal disease: Max 50 mg PO twice daily

X. Managing opioid side effects

  A. Constipation: All patients on opioids should have a preventive bowel regimen program in place. See Constipation on page 56.

  B. Nausea and vomiting: Occurs in approximately 25% of patients and usually short-lived, resolving in 3–7 days. Options include opioid rotation or decreasing dose. Medications to consider include haloperidol (first-line if mild–moderate), metoclopramide, prochlorperazine, scopolamine, and ondansetron (for severe symptoms). See Nausea and Vomiting on page 65.

  C. Delirium: Low risk unless elderly, attempt opioid rotation with a lower dose, may add low dose of haloperidol routinely. See Delirium on page 72.

  D. Myoclonus: Seen with chronic opioid usage and is unpredictable. Likely due to accumulation of toxic metabolites and increases with dehydration or with abnormal electrolytes. Treatment involves first correcting dehydration and replacing electrolytes, then opioid rotation with a lower dose. Consider clonazepam 0.5 mg PO twice daily or lorazepam 1 mg po q 8 h around the clock or midazolam infusion if severe. Other options include baclofen 5 mg PO twice daily.

  E. Opioid-induced hyperalgesia. Increasing sensitivity to various stimuli and increasing allodynia. Consider if increased moaning/pain despite intensive opioid escalation. Options include opioid rotation and ketamine.

  F. Overdose

    1. Diagnose with respiratory rate <8/min, shallow respirations, myoclonic twitching, constricted pupils, flaccid muscles, and/or cold/clammy skin. If awakens to voice or light touch, patient is sleeping, not overdosed. Note that in actively dying patients, apnea is typically due to brain stem dysfunction and not to opioid overdose (i.e., avoid naloxone if actively dying).

2. Naloxone: Stop opioid, dilute 0.4 mg/mL in 9 mL saline (i.e., 40 mcg/mL) and give 1 mL (0.04 mg) IV q 1 min until partial reversal noted and repeat until able to resume opioid at lower dosage. If no improvement after 0.8 mg total, consider other etiology such as benzodiazepines or stroke. Observe at least 4 hours for most opioids; if methadone overdose may need continuous naloxone infusion.

G. Pruritus: due to histamine release, can rotate to fentanyl if severe. Consider also ondansetron and naloxone.

H. Respiratory depression: Occurs rarely, can safely relieve dyspnea without causing respiratory depression.
   1. If easily arousable and respiratory rate >6/minute, can avoid administering an opioid antagonist.
   2. If pupils are not constricted and react to light, there is little chance of respiratory depression by increasing opioid dosage.
   3. Remember that a difficult to arouse level of sedation precedes respiratory depression

I. Sedation: Common initially and subsides in 2–5 days after steady dosing. Can be due to accumulated exhaustion and insomnia and patient catching up on sleep (these patients are easily arousable). Consider opioid rotation, decreased dose, or stimulants if prolonged symptoms. See Fatigue on page 83.

J. Addiction: Using despite harm, where increasing dose does not increase quality of life. A disease characterized by compulsive use of a substance despite physical or psychological harm to self or others.
   • Suggestive behaviors include frequent lost/stolen medications or altering opioid formulations, stealing money for medications, prescription fraud (such as forging or attempting to get multiple prescriptions from any source), selling medications or obtaining sex for medications.

K. Abuse: The intentional self-administration of a medication for a nonmedical purpose (such as to obtain a high)

L. Pseudoaddiction: Addictive-like behaviors that are iatrogenic and result from inadequate prescribing of analgesics.
   1. Behaviors include taking someone else's pain medications, aggressively complaining for more meds, worrying about changing meds, or doctor shopping. Frequently hoard meds to avoid running out.
   2. Will want to decrease dose if side effects increase.
   3. Behaviors cease when pain is controlled; quality of life improves as pain is better controlled.

M. Physical dependence (leading to withdrawal): Result of physically adapting to a medication such that withdrawal symptoms (diaphoresis, tachycardia, and nausea) occur when discontinued

N. Tolerance: Result of a biological process that leads to the need for increasing amounts of medication to achieve the same effect (this need is not indicative of addiction by itself)

ADJUVANTS

I. **NMDA antagonists**
   A. Dextromethorphan: Commonly used as an antitussive, has been found to be helpful in neuropathic pain in some patients (diabetic or posttrauma) at doses of 30–90 mg/day. High doses have been utilized (up to 270-mg single dose) but limited by lightheadedness and degree of metabolism (active metabolite has the analgesic effect). No improvement noted in postherpetic neuralgia patients.
   B. Methadone (see Methadone section on page 96)
   C. Ketamine: Utilize for analgesia in opioid-resistant pain, intractable neuropathic pain, allodynia, and hyperalgesia.
      1. Examples include severe bone pain/pathological fracture, spinal cord compression, tenesmus, and ischemic or phantom limb pain.
      2. Half-life is 1–3 h, up to 12 for active metabolite norketamine.
      3. Side effects include dysphoria, nausea, highly visual dreams or nightmares, excessive secretions, and psychomotor retardation/sedation. May decrease total opioid requirements therefore monitor for respiratory depression risk (consider decreasing or discontinuing long-acting opioids and switch to immediate-acting opioids when initiating ketamine).
         a. Psychomimetic side effects can be controlled with haloperidol (consider routine dosing) and/or benzodiazepines (consider routine dosing, for example lorazepam 0.5–1 mg IV q 4–8 hours).
      4. Based on anesthesia literature (10–20 times higher dosing) avoid ketamine in patients with neurological impairment, seizure disorder, hyperthyroidism, porphyria, or intracranial hypertension; caution in those with uncontrolled hypertension or heart failure, or if prior stroke.
      5. Dosing
         a. PO: Start 10–25 mg PO q 8 h, max 0.5–1 mg/kg q 8 h (can utilize IV formulation orally—onset 30 min, lasts 4–12 hours); oral can be more potent than IV route as first-pass metabolism converts to active metabolite norketamine; titrate by 20–30% every 3 days, decrease interval if end-of-dose failure noted

      b. SQ: 10–25 mg (0.2–0.5 mg/kg) ×1 prior to painful bedside procedures.

      c. IV: 0.1–0.2 mg/kg/h (onset 15 min). No loading dose. Monitor closely (hourly vitals ×24 h for initiation or dose changes, then at least twice daily once at steady dose). Titrate q 8–12 h until pain controlled.

         i. Some patients may need only pulse treatment and not need to transition to oral ketamine, but others may need ongoing treatment via ketamine PCA (demand dose example would be 0.08 mg/kg q 30 min).

    6. When converting IV to oral ketamine, use 1:1 conversion but stepwise over 2–3 days, note oral ketamine is more potent so may need lower total daily dose

  D. Levorphanol (see Levorphanol section on page 92)

II. Bisphosphonates/osteoclast inhibitors

  A. Most used in multiple myeloma and breast cancer with bone metastasis

    1. Lesser pain relief in lung, GI, and prostate cancers

  B. To decrease risk of jaw necrosis, ensure good dental hygiene, may need calcium/vitamin D supplementation to prevent hypocalcemia if using long-term

  C. 50–70% achieve 30% pain reduction in 1 week, duration is up to 12 weeks, but typically repeated monthly; treat flu-like syndrome with acetaminophen

  D. Pamidronate 90 mg IV over 2–4 h q 3–4 weeks (50% response rate within 1–2 weeks), common side effect is flu-like syndrome in first 48 h

  E. Zoledronic acid: IV over 15 min q 3–4 weeks (renal dose)

    1. GFR >60: 4 mg; 50–60:3.5; 40–49: 3.3; 30–39: 3

  F. Calcitonin: Not well studied, avoid using for bone pain

III. Corticosteroids

  A. Pain from inflammation at any site (bone, brain, spine, liver)

  B. Provide GI tract and thrush prophylaxis, watch sugars, watch for edema/fluid retention, and provide standard delirium precautions

  C. When tapering: if on <2 weeks (none), 2–4 weeks (rapid taper over days), >4 weeks (slow taper days to weeks)

  D. Drugs

    1. Dexamethasone: 4–8 mg PO qam (long T ½).

    2. Methylprednisolone: 16–32 mg PO two to three times per day

    3. Prednisone: 20–30 mg PO two to three times per day

IV. Antidepressants (neuropathic pain)

  A. Amitriptyline: 10–150 mg PO at bedtime

  B. Nortriptyline: 10–50 mg PO at bedtime

  C. Doxepin: 10–50 mg PO at bedtime

  D. Imipramine: 10–150 mg PO at bedtime

    E. Desipramine: 10–150 mg PO at bedtime

    F. Trazodone: 25–150 mg PO at bedtime

    G. Venlafaxine XR: 37.5–225 mg PO daily

    H. Duloxetine: 60 mg PO daily

V. Antispasmodics/muscle relaxants

    A. Use extra caution in geriatric patients.

    B. Baclofen: 5–20 mg PO three times per day

    C. Cyclobenzaprine: 5–10 mg PO three times per day or 15–30 mg ER PO daily

    D. Carisoprodol: 250–350 mg PO three times per day and at bedtime (up to 2–3 weeks)

    E. Methocarbamol: 1500 mg PO four times per day or 1g IV q 8 h (up to 3 days for acute muscle spasm)

    F. Clonidine: 0.1–0.3 mg PO two times per day (alpha-2 agonist)

    G. Tizanidine: at bedtime to twice daily (alpha-2 agonist, less hypotension than clonidine; consider for opioid-refractory neuropathic pain)

      • Starting dose: 2–4 mg PO q 8 h up to 36 mg/day

        a. Caution if creatinine clearance <25 or if hepatic impairment

VI. Anticonvulsant medications (neuropathic pain)

    A. Carbamazepine (numerous side effects, follow drug levels): 100 mg PO q 12 h up to 1200 mg/day (titrate weekly)

    B. Clonazepam: 0.5 mg PO two times per day

    C. Gabapentin: Start 100–300 mg/day, titrate up to 3600 mg/day. Dose q 8–12 h. Titrate every 1–3 days, slower in elderly (e.g., 300 mg PO at bedtime ×2 days, then 300 mg PO two times per day ×2 days, then 600 mg PO two times per day ×2 days, then 600 mg PO three times per day ×2 days, and so on [usual effective dose is 900–3600 mg/day])

      • Renal dosing: Max daily dose for CrCl 30–60 ml/min is 1400 mg/day. For CrCl 16–30 mL/min, 700 mg/day. For CrCl <15 mL/min, <300 mg daily to every other day if CrCl 7.5 mL/min. Tolerance to side effects of sedation, confusion, dizziness, and ataxia commonly develop, after a few days if medication able to be continued.

    D. Lamotrigine (Lamictal): If not on other anticonvulsants, start 25 mg PO daily × 2 weeks, then increase 25 mg q 1–2 weeks, up to 200 mg po q 12 h

    E. Oxcarbazepine (Trileptal): Fewer side effects than carbamazepine, caution hyponatremia; 300 mg PO twice daily and titrate up to 2400 mg/day

    F. Phenytoin (Dilantin): Follow free or albumin-corrected total drug levels; consider IV loading (10–15 mg/kg or if myoclonus/seizure present 15–20 mg/kg at max rate of 50 mg/minute) and monitor

pain or symptom response. If good response, transition to oral regimen (short acting is three times per day dosing, usual range 300–600 mg/day). Oral loading is 15–20 mg/kg.

G. Pregabalin (Lyrica): Caution euphoria, 25–50 mg PO q 12 h up to 150–300 mg q 12 h (titrate over 1 week)

H. Topiramate: 25 mg PO daily, titrate 25–50 mg weekly up to 400 mg daily (given twice daily)

I. Valproate (Depakote): Follow drug levels, 250 mg PO/IV at bedtime up to 60 mg/kg/day (divided q 8–12 h, max 1200 mg/day)

VII. Anesthetics (neuropathic pain): Lidocaine

A. 5% transdermal patch (700 mg in a 10 × 14-cm patch) or 2–5% gel/ointment q 6 h.
   1. Patch Studied up to 12 h/day, but often needed up to 24 h/day for pain relief in some patients
   2. Less than 5% of the lidocaine is absorbed systemically, can utilize up to 3 patches
   3. Avoid in liver failure

B. SQ/IV
   1. Half-life is 1.5–2 h, time to analgesia is 1–45 min
   2. Loading: 2 mg/kg over 20 min; infuse: 1–3 mg/kg/h
   3. Follow levels based on side-effect symptoms below, if needed/feasible can confirm with serum levels: 8 h after start/adjustments then weekly, goal level: 2–6 mcg/mL or mg/L
   4. Side effects (can approximate level in mcg/mL based on symptoms):
      a. lightheadedness (1 mcg/mL)
      b. perioral numbness (2)
      c. metallic taste (3)
      d. tinnitus (5–6)
      e. If the following adverse effects develop, stop immediately: blurred vision (6), myoclonus (8), seizures (10), bradycardia (20–25), cardiovascular shock (>25)
   5. If responds, consider oral mexiletine
      a. Mexiletine: 150 mg PO two to four times per day

VIII. Cannabinoids

A. Consider for neuropathic pain in cancer patients refractory to opioids and other adjuvants.

B. Caution due to dizziness, somnolence, and dry mouth.

C. Dronabinol 2.5 PO once or twice daily

D. Nabilone 0.5–1 mg PO at bedtime up to 3 mg two times per day

IX. Topical agents:

A. Capsaicin cream 0.025–0.075% three to four times per day

B. Diclofenac patch/cream/gel

C. Doxepin cream

D. EMLA cream

PROCEDURES

I. **Trigger-point injections:** 1–3 mL of 1% lidocaine or 0.25% bupivacaine directly into painful muscle site

II. **Nerve blocks:** Nonneurolytic (analgesic) or neurolytic (anesthetic). Side effects result from loss of sympathetic tone (such as hypotension and diarrhea due to unopposed parasympathetic activity) or injury such as paraplegia. Consider utilizing if prognosis <3–6 months as decreased effectiveness can be seen with repeat blocks

   A. Abdominal viscera (distal third of esophagus to transverse colon, liver, biliary tract, adrenals, and mesentery): Celiac plexus/splanchnic nerve

   B. Facial: Gasserian ganglion block

   C. Pelvic viscera (urogenital, descending colon to rectum): Superior hypogastric plexus

   D. Rib fractures: intercostal blocks

   E. Rectal pain (i.e., tenesmus), perineum: Ganglion impar block

   F. Shoulder pain: Brachial plexus or suprascapular block

III. **Epidural**

   A. Morphine starting dose is 10% of the daily oral morphine equivalent; can utilize patient-controlled epidural analgesia (PCEA) with lockouts from 10 minutes (fentanyl) to 60–90 minutes (morphine); lockout about 15 minutes for local anesthetics

   B. Epidural steroids should be considered for an acute herniated disc with radiculopathy.

IV. **Intrathecal (IT): Side effects include risk of CSF leak, infections, and headache; if prognosis <3 months consider an external pump, if >3 months utilize an implanted pump**

   A. Baclofen

   B. Morphine starting dose: 1% of the daily oral morphine equivalent, or 100 mg IV morphine is 1 mg IT morphine.

   C. Ziconotide (for patients refractory to other therapies including intrathecal morphine): Avoid if history of psychosis, risk of neurological, or psychiatric impairment.

RADIOPHARMACEUTICAL THERAPIES

I. Bone-seeking radioisotopes (via nuclear medicine department) for multifocal bone pain from osteoblastic lesions.

II. Patient not a candidate or failed standard radiotherapy, opioids, or other adjuvants.

  III. Has >12 weeks prognosis, and (due to high-risk of myelosuppression) should have WBC ≥3K and platelets >60–100K, normal renal function, not pregnant, and not expected to need future myelosuppressive chemotherapy).

  IV. Analgesia begins in 60–80% of patients within 1–2 weeks and lasts 2–6 months. Bone marrow recovery occurs in 8–12 weeks; 10–20% have a pain flare within the first week that may be predictive of a positive response.

  V. Verify dose using a radioactivity calibration system immediately before administration.

  VI. Drink and void well after treatment.

  VII. Drugs.

    A. Strontium-89 (Metastron) IV: 148 megabecquerel (4 millicurie) or weight-based at 1.5–2.2 megabecquerel (40–60 microcurie)/kg over 1–2 minutes; repeat as needed q 90 days

    B. Samarium-153 (Quadramet) IV: 37 megabecquerels (1 millicurie)/kg over 1 minute

SPECIFIC CONDITIONS

  I. **Visceral pain:** Anticholinergics (scopolamine, oxybutynin for bladder spasms), steroids, benzodiazepines, octreotide

  II. **Bone pain:** NSAIDs, glucocorticoids (dexamethasone), bisphosphonates, radiotherapy

    A. Vertebral collapse: If pain refractory to standard treatment and prognosis > few months, consider vertebroplasty or kyphoplasty

  III. **Cirrhosis:**

    A. Safest is fentanyl

    B. Caution (utilized reduced dosage/intervals): morphine, oxycodone, and hydromorphone

    C. Consider: Baclofen (may also assist with maintaining alcohol abstinence)

  IV. **Chronic kidney disease:**

    A. Severe to end-stage chronic kidney disease: Safest is fentanyl or methadone. Hydromorphone with caution (should be tolerated with effective dialysis for ESRD patients).

    B. Moderate to severe chronic kidney disease: hydromorphone, oxycodone with caution (reduced dosage and frequency)

    C. Mild to moderate chronic kidney disease: morphine, hydromorphone. Consider reducing dosage and frequency as renal function declines.

COMPLEMENTARY THERAPIES

   I. **Biofeedback:** Find a practitioner at the Biofeedback Certification Institute of America (www.bcia.org)

  II. **Deep breathing:** Exhale when you anticipate a painful stimulus; breathe deeply, slowly, and consciously; lightly stroke the area of pain to associate the technique with relief of pain

 III. **Exercise and stretching** (as possible with underlying condition)

 IV. **Massage therapy:** Find a practitioner at the American Massage Therapy Association (www.amtamassage.org)

  V. **Music therapy:** Find a practitioner at the American Music Therapy Association (www.musictherapy.org)

 VI. **Prayer and meditation**

9 ■ RESPIRATORY

CHRONIC COUGH

I. Background information
A. Response to irritation of cough receptors located in the upper and lower respiratory tract, esophagus, diaphragm, stomach, and even pericardium
1. Signals transmitted via the vagus nerve to the medulla.
2. Most common etiologies include postnasal drip (upper airway cough syndrome), asthma, and gastroesophageal reflux.
3. Other etiologies include postinfection, medications (ACE-inhibitors), chronic bronchitis, or cancer.
4. May also be due to clinically silent aspiration.
5. Severe coughing spells may result in rib fractures.

II. Evaluation
A. History and physical to identify or eliminate the previously listed common causes.
- If appropriate, referrals to speech therapists (swallow testing), head and neck, or pulmonary specialists should be considered.

III. Management
A. Treatments specific for suspected etiologies should be attempted.
- May need to treat all suspected etiologies simultaneously
B. If no specific etiology identified or cough is disabling, the following agents should be considered:
1. Opioids:
   a. Codeine 10–30 mg PO q 4–6 h up to 120 mg/day)
   b. Morphine 5–10 mg slow release PO twice daily or 2.5–5 mg solution PO q 4–6 h
   c. Dextromethorphan 10–20 mg PO q 4–6 h or 30 mg PO q 6–8 h or 60 mg ER PO twice daily up to 120 mg/day
3. Benzonatate (Tessalon) 100 mg PO three times per day up to 200 mg PO three times per day (lung/pleura stretch receptor anesthetic), consider using along with guaifenesin and/or with opioids (advanced cancer patients).
4. Thalidomide: 100–400 mg PO daily has been utilized for idiopathic pulmonary fibrosis patients.
5. Inhaled lidocaine: For refractory chronic cough due to endobronchial malignancy, try 5 mL of 2% lidocaine via nebulizer q 4 h and titrated as needed up to 300 mg daily.
   a. Consider administering after albuterol to reduce risk of bronchospasm; avoid oral intake for 1 hour after treatment completed to reduce risk of aspiration or accidental injury to oropharynx.
6. Consider trials of inhaled glucocorticoids or ipratropium bromide.

DYSPNEA

I. **Background information**
   A. Also known as breathlessness
   B. Common source of suffering and dread defined as "a subjective experience of breathing discomfort"

II. **Evaluation**
   A. Dyspnea is subjective, so patient history is the gold standard.
      1. Patients may describe feeling like they are being smothered, suffocating, unable to breathe, feeling tight, or unable to stop thinking about breathing.
      2. Dyspnea does not correlate well with hypoxia, hypercarbia, or tachypnea.
      3. Like pain, episodes may be periodic, occurring several times a day rather than constantly.
      4. Similar to total pain, total dyspnea involves assessing for physical (cancer, effusions, hypoxia/hypercarbia, drug toxicity, ascites, constipation), psychological (anxiety, coping), social (finances, family), and spiritual (meaning) components, and providing appropriate interventions for each contributing etiology.
      5. Several scales exist such as the cancer dyspnea scale, respiratory distress observation scale (for patients unable to self-report), standard numerical 0–10 scale, and the Edmonton symptom assessment scale.
         a. Important to use the same scale for follow-up to determine how effective interventions have been

III. **Management**
   A. Treat the underlying cause of dyspnea if possible and consistent with the patient's goals of care.
      1. If early in the dying process and anemia is identified as the cause, blood transfusions may relieve dyspnea and provide a sense of energy for several weeks.
      2. Thoracentesis/pleurodesis, bronchoscopy (stents, mucous plugs), palliative chemotherapy or radiotherapy, and noninvasive or invasive assisted ventilation may be indicated depending on the patient's goals of care and the risks/benefits in relation to prognosis (even if underlying terminally illness).
   B. Specific medications.
      1. Antibiotics if dyspnea related to infectious etiology
      2. Benzodiazepines if patient also has an anxiety component, if terminal dyspnea continuous regimen may be required
      3. Bronchodilators if bronchospasm present
      4. Corticosteroids—chronic obstructive pulmonary disease, asthma, SVC syndrome, lymphangitis

5. Diuretics—heart failure, fluid overload, some effusions.
   a. Decrease burden of incoming fluids as appropriate if contributing to fluid overload and dyspnea (such as IVFs, tube feedings, TPN).
6. Nitrates for heart failure.
7. Opioids (e.g., morphine, hydromorphone, fentanyl)—via any route.
   a. Example: Morphine 5 mg IR PO q 4 h as needed for dyspnea, then convert to long-acting formulation.
   b. Titrate rapidly if terminal dyspnea present, continuous regimen may be required.
   c. Unclear if nebulized morphine helpful routinely for most patients in part due to possible bronchospasm from histamine release. Can utilize 2.5 to 10 mg of IV morphine (preservative free most studied) in 2 mL normal saline with 2–4 mg of dexamethasone (to reduce bronchospasm risk) as a nebulizer treatment.
8. Oxygen: May be helpful if patient is hypoxic on room air.
9. Helium + oxygen mixture; May be helpful if tracheal obstruction (stridor) present.
10. Theophylline is controversial for use in chronic obstructive pulmonary disease patients. Generally avoid as no help for exacerbations. If used as a 3rd-line agent (after anticholinergics and beta-2 agonists) for chronic, stable patients, some patients may report improved dyspnea (goal serum level 8–12 mcg/mL). Higher seizure risk if hypoalbuminemia. Risk of increased nausea, tremors, and arrhythmias.

C. Nonmedical interventions.
1. Positioning: Keep head of bed elevated, lean forward, or knees toward chest.
2. Teach pursed-lip breathing: Inhale slowly via nose, exhale via "kissed lips."
3. Keep air flowing with a fan or open windows, or via nasal cannula if provides relief.
4. Family presence.
5. Relaxation therapy.

HICCUPS

I. Background information
A. Hiccups, or singultus, are involuntary contractions of the diaphragm and intercostal muscles.
B. A bout can last up to 48 hours.
   • Persistent if >48 h up to 1 month, and considered intractable if >1 month
C. Possible etiologies.
1. GI irritation such as distension (overeating, tube feeds), reflux, sudden temperature changes, and alcohol can lead to hiccups.

2. Anxiety can also contribute.
3. Persistent or intractable hiccups often seen with drug use (dexamethasone, diazepam, barbiturates); disorders involving the CNS, GI tract, or thorax; and electrolyte imbalances (uremia, hypocalcemia, hyponatremia, and hyperglycemia)

II. Evaluation

A. Evaluate for underlying trigger or etiology.
- May include imaging and blood work to identify trigger

III. Management

A. Nonmedical
1. Valsalva (holding breath under forced expiration) or holding breath
2. Sipping cold water slowly
3. Swallow teaspoon of dry sugar
4. Press on the eyeballs

B. Medical
1. Baclofen: 5–20 mg PO q 8–12 h, use lower doses in elderly
2. Chlorpromazine (first-line): 10–25 mg PO/IM q 6–8 h, titrate up to 50 mg PO/IM q 6–8 h for up to 10 days. Stop 1 day after cessation of hiccups. If needed 25–50 mg IV via slow IV infusion (i.e., in 500–1000 mL NS and patient supine to reduce hypotension). Avoid in elderly dementia patients.
3. Gabapentin: 300–400 mg PO q 8 h.
4. Haloperidol: 1–5 mg PO/SQ q 8 h.
5. Metoclopramide: 10–20 mg PO/SQ q 6–8 hours up to 10 days.
6. Phenytoin: 200 mg slow IV push, then 300 mg PO daily. May be effective for patients with underlying CNS etiology.
7. Steroid trial.

ORAL SECRETIONS

I. Background information

A. Excessive oral secretions are most distressing to family and friends near the end of life ("death rattle").
- Less so to the patient

B. Can be exacerbated by excessive fluid intake (oral, IVF, tube feeds, TPN).
- Both oral and bronchial secretions may respond well to anticholinergics, but secretions from heart failure do not respond well to these interventions.
  a. Consider maximizing opioid use and gentle diuresis for those situations.

II. Evaluation

A. Identify degree of distress to patient and family.
- Explain this is a normal sound and often not distressing to the patient and can be likened in some cases to snoring.

III. **Management**
  A. Nonmedical
    1. Positioning to a lateral decubitus position
    2. Suctioning only if choking present or if absolutely needed to decrease patient distress
      a. Ineffective in long term, may exacerbate distress
  B. Medical
    1. Glycopyrrolate (first-line, does not cross the blood-brain barrier): 0.4–2 mg PO/SL q 4 h, 0.2–0.4 mg SQ q 4 h, 0.4–1.2 mg/day continuous IV infusion
    2. Atropine: 0.4 mg SQ q 2–4 h, 2 mg via nebulizer q 2–4 h, 1–2% ophthalmic drops (2–10 drops SL q 2–4 h), 0.4 mg IV q 1–2 h
    3. Hyoscyamine: 0.125–0.25 mg PO/SL q 2–4 h or 0.25–0.5 mg SQ q 2–4 h
    4. Scopolamine: 1.5-mg transdermal patch, 1–3 patches q 72 h
      a. May take up to 12 hours to start working

PLEURAL EFFUSIONS

I. **Background information**
  A. Recurrent pleural effusions commonly lead to dyspnea, orthopnea, coughing, and chest pain.
  B. Depending on prognosis, treatment should be aimed at the underlying cause.
    • If due to malignancy, pleurodesis or permanent drainage catheter should be considered.

II. **Evaluation**
  A. Etiology of pleural effusion should be identified to help guide treatment.
    1. Systemic causes (transudative) include heart failure, cirrhosis, and nephrotic syndrome.
    2. Local causes (exudative) include infections, malignancy, autoimmune disorders, and pulmonary embolism.

III. **Management**
  A. Treat underlying systemic etiology if possible.
  B. Repeated thoracentesis if rare can be considered, but less overall risk if pleurodesis performed or indwelling catheter placed (for home drainage as needed).
  C. Pleurodesis options include doxycycline (pain, fever), bleomycin (fever), and talc powder (pain, fever, may lead to residual loculated effusions).

TERMINAL EXTUBATION PROTOCOLS

I. **Background information**
   A. When considered, all plans should be reviewed with goals to maximize patient comfort.
      - All present should be updated on what signs and symptoms they may see including ongoing "breathing on their own" for minutes, hours, or even days until natural death occurs.

II. **Evaluation**
   A. Review to make sure patient's wishes or goals of care are being honored.

III. **Management**
   A. Protocols should ensure maximal patient and family comfort.
      1. Remove restraints, discontinue alarms and monitoring equipment, and allow space for family (minimizing distractions to family).
      2. Utilize opioids and benzodiazepines to achieve moderate-to-deep sedation.
      3. Consider anticholinergics to reduce secretions.
      4. Discontinue vasopressors, TPN, antibiotics, and other sources of excess fluid or interventions that might increase dyspnea, pain, anxiety, and/or prolong the natural dying process.
      5. Once comfortable, set ventilator to room air and ensure comfort, then decrease PEEP to ≤10 and ensure patient remains comfortable, then remove ventilator support with ongoing titration of opioids and benzodiazepines as needed to prevent tachypnea, tachycardia, grimacing, agitation, or any other signs of distress.
         a. If patient can breathe independently, ensure other comfort medications have been ordered (antiemetics, antipyretics).
         b. O_2 via nasal cannula should only be provided low flow if it relieves distress (often times it does not).
            i. High-flow O_2 or O_2 via mask often increases end-of-life dyspnea.

MALODOROUS FUNGATING WOUNDS

I. **Background information**
  A. Malignant fungating wounds can result from primary skin cancers (basal cell, squamous cell, and melanoma) or secondarily via direct extension or metastatic spread of other cancers.
  B. May fail to heal due to progressive cancer despite interventions.
    • Can result in pain, infections, profuse drainage (exudates or bleeding), strong odor (from anaerobic bacteria), and social distress and isolation

II. **Evaluation**
  A. Evaluate anatomical location, degree of tissue damage, size, degree of drainage or bleeding, and findings such as tenderness and odor.
  B. Consider biopsy if needed.
  C. Optimize patient's nutritional and hydration status if possible depending on underlying illness, prognosis, and goals of care.
  D. Evaluate degree of psychosocial distress wound is causing.

III. **Management**
  A. Basics
    1. Keep wound or ulcer bed moist by cleansing and providing regular dressing changes (increasing autolytic debridement and minimizing infections).
    2. Cleanse with warmed normal saline (can use 30–60-mL syringe with 18–20-gauge angiocath). Cold NS causes pain.
      a. Avoid saline "wet to dry" orders (dressing removal leads to bleeding and pain).
      b. Soak off dressing with warm normal saline.
      c. Consider topical lidocaine to reduce pain.
    3. Obtain wound care specialist consultation for assistance.
    4. Aim for twice-a-day dressings for home use to decrease caregiver burden.
  B. Wound pain
    1. Morphine: 0.1% (1 mg:1 mL ratio with cream, ointment, or solution) or 0.5% (5 mg:1 mL ratio with cream, ointment, or solution) q 24 h
      a. Example: Mix 10 mg of morphine sulfate injection (10 mg/mL) in 8 grams of IntraSite gel. Cover wound with 5–10 mL of gel and loosely dress with gauze, change 1–3 ×/day as needed (mixture stable up to 28 days).

    2. 2–4% lidocaine spray solution: Make by mixing 5 mL of 1 mEq/mL sodium bicarbonate (to buffer) with 45 mL of 2 or 4% lidocaine.

      a. Use within 1 week, max 200 mg/24 h.

C. Odor (predominately due to anaerobic bacteria)

  1. Debride necrotic tissue.

  2. Apply an agent to reduce bacterial load or odors.

    a. Silver dressings: once or twice daily

    b. Metronidazole: 1% gel (or compounded from crushed tablets) once or twice daily for 2 weeks (repeat as needed)

    c. Cadexomer iodine (Iodosorb, Iodoflex): 3×/week for up to 3 months

    d. Consider irradiated honey (controls odor and may reduce tumor size)

    e. For yeast, utilize clotrimazole

    f. For pseudomonas, utilize diluted acetic acid

    g. Activated carbon (charcoal) dressing

    h. Mesalt dressing

    i. Curcumin ointment (from turmeric)

    j. Baking soda in between dressing layers

    k. Consider systemic metronidazole 500 mg PO/IV q 6–8 h (caution nausea)

    l. If determined to be irreversibly nonhealing, consider topical povidone-iodine (i.e., Betadine); pretreat with an anesthetic if needed to reduce pain. Apply as a topical solution as paint on the wound.

  3. Social isolation (due to odor)

    a. Ensure adequate room ventilation.

    b. Utilize activated charcoal or basket of charcoal briquettes or kitty litter (i.e., in tray under bed).

    c. Burn candles.

    d. Bowls of cider vinegar, vanilla, or coffee grounds.

    e. Avoid fragrances and perfumes as often poorly tolerated, but air freshener sprays or peppermint may be tolerated.

D. Drainage

  1. Exudates: If very heavy, consider a drainable ostomy or wound collection device.

  2. Absorbent foam dressings (covered by a gauze pad).

  3. Alginate dressings.

  4. Polysaccharide dextranomer beads.

  5. Cadexomer iodine dressings.

E. Bleeding

  1. Alginate packing

  2. Topical thromboplastin (100 units/mL)

  3. Silver nitrate

  4. Cautery

  5. Epinephrine

PRESSURE ULCERS

I. **Background information**
    A. Pressure ulcers are due to lack of adequate blood supply as a result of direct pressure that ruptures the muscle membranes.
        1. Skin receives ⅓ of the body's blood supply.
        2. Friction can damage the top epidermal layer, and shear forces can damage deeper layers contributing to even greater damage from pressure.
        3. Moisture and heat can also contribute to skin breakdown.

II. **Evaluation**
    A. Document at minimum these 4 items:
        1. Date noticed
        2. Location
        3. Stage, size, and description of wound bed
        4. Pain and/or odor
    B. Stages
        1. Nonblanchable erythema of the epidermis, but the majority of the damage has likely already occurred in deeper layers
        2. Abrasion, blister, or shallow crater (partial thickness involving epidermis +/− dermis)
        3. Deep ulcer: Full thickness ulcer down to the fascia (subcutaneous tissue)
        4. Ulcer goes down to muscle, bone, tendon, or joint capsule; may have sinus tract tunneling.
        5. Unstageable: Likely stage 3 or 4, but unknown as ulcer is covered by slough and/or eschar
    C. Deep tissue injury: Injury frequently from intense pressure and shear forces
        1. Purple or maroon area of intact skin; tissue is painful, mushy or firm, and warmer or cooler than adjacent tissue.
        2. Evolution may be rapid, exposing multiple layers even with optimal treatment.
    D. Kennedy terminal ulcer: A result of a patient actively dying with multiorgan failure (the skin is another organ that is failing)
        1. Often a sign of impending death (within 8–24 hours) and sometimes looks like a butterfly, pear, or horseshoe (usually sacral area, large, changes from red to yellow to black, with irregular borders)
        2. Begins as a stage 2 (blister) and rapidly progresses to stage 3–4
        3. Thought to be due to expected loss of blood flow when approaching death, which likely manifests itself in areas of greatest pressure
        4. Exacerbated by less movement and turning when attempting to maximize comfort during the dying process

III. Management

A. Support surfaces such as static or alternating air or water mattress overlays (moderate risk), low air loss or microclimate management beds (high risk or current ulceration), or air-fluidized beds (maximum pressure relief).

B. Avoid saline wet-to-dry dressings.

C. Necrotic tissue ideally should be debrided, but should not be attempted if patient close to dying or with poor vascular supply to limbs as wound will never heal.

D. Turn the patient off of the pressure ulcer, side to side turning if ulcer on sacrum, limit sitting if ulcers on ischium.

E. Wound care specialist evaluation.

F. Improve intake of protein and calories if possible.

G. Ulcer management.

    1. Stage 1 ulcers: OpSite and Tegaderm

    2. For deeper but clean wounds: DuoDERM, Comfeel, Tegasorb, and Restore

    3. For wounds with significant drainage: IntraSite, Elasto-Gel, ClearSite, Aquasorb, Kaltostat, Sorbsan, Lyofoam, Allevyn, Nu-Derm, and Flexzan

PRURITUS

I. Background information

A. Pruritus (itching) is having the feeling of needing to scratch.

B. Etiologies.

    1. Peripheral (urticarial)

    2. Neuropathic (herpes zoster)

    3. Central/systemic

        a. Cholestasis/liver failure

        b. Renal failure

        c. Histamine or serotonin release (can be opioid-induced)

C. Severe pruritus can result in insomnia and skin excoriation.

II. Evaluation

A. Obtain a drug history, relieving/exacerbating factors, and skin examination.

B. If appropriate, obtain a CBC, ESR, thyroid, and renal/liver function tests.

C. Dermatologist evaluation for possible biopsy should be considered.

D. Possible etiologies.

    1. Most common is xerosis (dry skin).

    2. Other peripheral etiologies include scabies, insect bites, candida infection, lice, eczema and urticaria, contact dermatitis, psoriasis, cancer lesions (metastatic or local), and paraneoplastic syndromes.

3. Systemic etiologies include thyroid disorders, carcinoid, uremia, cholestasis, iron deficiency, polycythemia vera, brain lesions (strokes, abscess, tumors), drug induced (opioids, aspirin, allergic reactions), chronic lymphocytic leukemia, and lymphomas.

III. Management

A. General treatment options
1. Mild pruritus: Calamine lotion, and/or 0.5–4% menthol creams, oatmeal baths (avoid hot water in bath)
2. Moderate to severe pruritis
   a. Inflammatory etiology
      i. Topical steroid ointments (systemic steroids if refractory).
      ii. NSAIDs include tacrolimus 0.03–0.1% ointment and pimecrolimus 1% cream.
      iii. Systemic agents include cyclosporine, azathioprine, and mycophenolate.
   b. Antihistamines: Consider combining traditional H1 blockers such as diphenhydramine 12.5–50 mg PO/SQ q 6 h or hydroxyzine 10–50 mg PO/SQ q 4 h with H2 blockers such as cimetidine
   c. Direct anesthetic with anesthetic creams: Pramoxine 1% cream or lotion twice daily, ethyl chloride spray, lidocaine 2.5% with prilocaine 2.5% cream (i.e., EMLA)
   d. SSRIs can be helpful (paroxetine, fluvoxamine, sertraline) as well as the TCA doxepin (10–75 mg PO at bedtime)
3. For severe refractory pruritus consider aprepitant (NK-1 antagonist)
B. Specific conditions
1. Dry skin: Moisturizing agents such as petroleum jelly or emollients immediately applied after cleansing using gentle soaps
2. Tumor-related pruritus
   a. H2 blockers (cimetidine): Up to 800 mg/24 h
   b. NSAIDs
   c. Cholestyramine (hematologic tumors)
   d. 5HT3 antagonists (ondansetron)
   e. SSRIs (paroxetine): 5–20 mg PO daily
   f. Mirtazapine: 7.5–15 mg PO at bedtime
   g. Dexamethasone: 4–8 mg PO daily
3. Uremia
   a. 5HT3 antagonists
   b. Opioid receptor antagonists (such as naltrexone 50–100 mg PO daily): Caution withdrawal, even if opioid-naïve due to endogenous opioids
   c. Cholestyramine: 4 g daily–6×/day up to 24 g/day total
   d. Thalidomide: 100 mg PO daily
   e. Phototherapy (UVB)

  f. Capsaicin cream: In 70% of patients for whom pruritus is localized, burning sensation with initial treatment can last up to 30 minutes and resolves within 3 weeks

   i. Pretreatment with a topical anesthetic may help.

  g. Mirtazapine: 7.5–15 mg po q pm

4. Cholestasis

  a. Relieving the obstruction is the most effective method (surgery, chemotherapy, biliary stent, high-dose dexamethasone)

  b. Opioid receptor antagonists: Naloxone, naltrexone 12.5–250 mg daily

  c. Cholestyramine: 4 g PO three times per day or charcoal if enough bile draining to GI tract

  d. Phototherapy (UVB)

  e. Rifampicin: 75 mg PO daily–150 mg PO twice daily

   i. Be aware of idiosyncratic side effects.

5. Neuropathic pruritus

  a. Topical anesthetics

  b. Gabapentin or pregabalin

  c. Capsaicin cream

6. Polycythemia vera

  a. Standard disease-modifying therapy first line

  b. Aspirin

  c. Paroxetine

  d. Cimetidine

  e. Psoralen + phototherapy (PUVA)

PART III: EMERGENCIES AND FURTHER READING

11 ■ EMERGENCIES

I. **Background information**
   A. Signs of approaching death may not be obvious to family members.
      1. Ensure caretakers have been instructed on what to expect as death approaches. Even with careful preparation, family members may still view this time as an emergency and seek emergency help.
      2. Providing brochures on what to expect and 24/7 contact information is helpful.
II. **Evaluation**
   A. 3 stages of actively dying
      1. Stage I (early active phase)
         a. Dysphagia (increasing aspiration risk)
         b. Terminal anorexia (force feeding/hydration increases nausea/vomiting, heart failure, ascites, and peripheral edema)
         c. Fatigue/drowsiness
         d. Weakness
         e. Emotional withdrawal
         f. Mild hypotension, tachy-/bradypnea, and tachy-/bradycardia
      2. Stage II (active phase; up to few days prior to death)
         a. Tachycardia (HR >120)
         b. Hypotension (<80/40)
         c. Cool extremities/cyanosis
         d. Oliguria (<500 mL/day)
         e. Bedbound
         f. Severe dysphagia
         g. Hyper-/hypothermia
         h. Cheyne-Stokes respirations
         i. Death rattle (can occur 1–3 days prior to death due to inability to clear secretions in the hypopharynx)
         j. Near comatose
         k. Terminal delirium
         l. Respirations by mandibular movement (RMM, or "O" sign)
         m. Flaccid pinna (earlobe falls to nape of neck when head turned to the side)
         n. Near death awareness (visual and auditory hallucinations)
      3. Stage III (imminent death; hours to 1–2 days prior to death)
         a. Increasing RMM (near 70% within 6 hours of death)
         b. increasing Cheyne-Stokes respirations with increasing apnea periods and rate decreasing to 4–6 breaths/minute

    c. Pulsus alternans (alternating strong/weak beats)

    d. Cool mandible

    e. Patellar mottling (knee mottling with reticular pattern)

    f. Increasing cyanosis (lips and fingers, 80% within 6 hours of death)

    g. Mottling

    h. Nasolabial fold drooping, relaxed forehead and face (appears angelic or very peaceful to some people)

    i. Neck hyperextension with tense sternocleidomastoid muscle (patient seems to look straight up)

    j. Loss of rectal tone

    k. Absent bowel sounds

    l. Kennedy terminal ulcer (can occur in <4 hours, rapid onset, may look like a butterfly, more an ischemic ulcer than a pressure ulcer)

    m. Loss of both radial pulses (near 90% death likely within 6 hours)

B. Death is expected within hours if patient has all 4 of the following:
1. Death rattle
2. RMM
3. Cyanosis/mottling
4. Loss of both radial pulses

III. Management

A. Normalize the signs of dying for caregivers.
- These signs are an expected and natural part of dying and should not be considered an emergency however may be perceived as such by family members who are not adequately prepared.
  a. It is difficult for family members and healthcare providers to see progressive hypotension and hypoxia and not want to intervene in the natural dying process.
  b. Provide education ahead of time on what to expect and discontinue routine vitals and minimize disturbances (e.g., can the patient be turned less frequently?).

ACUTE BLEEDING

I. Background information

A. Bleeding can be very traumatic for patient, family, and healthcare staff.
- If anticipated or high risk for bleeding, patients and family members should be made aware of the risk and have a management plan
  a. Those at highest risk include those with prior recurrent bleeding episodes (hemoptysis, hematemesis, hematuria, hematochezia, vaginal bleeding); those with large

head, neck, or lung tumors close to large blood vessels; those with liver failure; and those with suppressed bone marrow.

II. Evaluation

A. Identify goals of care to help guide workup (labs) and interventions (such as fluid resuscitation or transfusions) that may or may not be desired or indicated.

III. Management

A. Local measures
   1. If possible, especially if at home recommend to use or have available dark red or black towels and bedding (prior to an anticipated bleed).
   2. Reduce patient anxiety (lorazepam or midazolam).
   3. Apply pressure or packing (may include hemostatic agents); hemostatic dressings may be used.
   4. Consider single-dose radiotherapy (lung, rectum, vagina, head and neck, and bladder cancers).
   5. Inject sclerosing agents or consider laser coagulation (UGI tract, lungs, and bladder).
   6. Interventional radiology for arterial embolization (head and neck, lung, gynecological, and GI tract cancer patients).
   7. Surgical evaluation.

B. Systemic measures
   1. Vitamin K (liver disease or malnutrition): 2.5–10 mg SQ/PO daily.
   2. Octreotide: 50–100 micrograms SQ/IV once or twice daily up to 600 micrograms/day (GI tract bleeding).
   3. Antifibrinolytic agents.
      a. Tranexamic acid: 10 mg/kg IV q 6 h (infused over 1 hour)
      b. Aminocaproic acid: 4–5 g IV over 1 hour, then 1 g/hour for 8 hours or until bleeding stops (max daily dose 30 g)
         i. For severe thrombocytopenia, utilize 100 mg/kg IV dose (max 5 g) over 30–60 minutes, then 1 g/hour (up to 24 g/day)
   4. Platelet transfusions: Consider for symptom control of gum bleeding, epistaxis, painful hematomas, or continuous bleeding from GI/GU cancers.
   5. Packed red blood cells: Consider for severe symptomatic anemia.
   6. Fresh frozen plasma: Consider if needed to reverse oral anticoagulation.

ANAPHYLAXIS

I. **Background information**
   A. Anaphylaxis is a severe life-threatening allergic reaction to a trigger.
   - Triggers can be environmental or medications.

II. **Evaluation**
   A. Observe for rapid onset (minutes to several hours) of the following.
   1. Skin signs (hives, flushed, swollen lips)
   2. Mucosal changes (swollen tongue and uvula)
   3. Respiratory signs (wheezing, stridor, hypoxia)
   4. Cardiac signs (hypotension, syncope, incontinence)
   5. GI signs (vomiting)

III. **Management**
   A. Contact emergency services; short-term intubation may be required.
   B. Medication
   1. Epinephrine (1:1000 or 0.1%, which is 1 mg/mL) 0.3–0.5 mg IM to mid-anterolateral thigh, repeat q 5–15 min as needed.
      a. Should be given within 30 minutes of symptom onset
   2. For patients on beta-blockers, if not responding to epinephrine, utilize glucagon 1–5 mg IV over 5 minutes (caution vomiting).
   3. Consider utilizing diphenhydramine 25–50 mg IV AFTER epinephrine if needed to relieve itch and hives.

CARDIAC TAMPONADE

I. **Background information**
   A. When fluid accumulates within the pericardial sac and pressure increases, it can result in cardiac tamponade.
   - Fluid may accumulate due to infections, radiation, neoplasms, post-MI, pericarditis, trauma (such as CPR), autoimmune disorders, drugs, uremia, and hypothyroidism.

II. **Evaluation**
   A. Patients may report worsening dyspnea, chest pain, lower extremity edema, and fatigue.
   B. Examination may reveal sinus tachycardia, markedly elevated jugular venous pressure, pulsus paradoxus (systolic drop of >10 mm Hg on inspiration), and hypotension.
   - Confirm by echocardiography.

III. **Management**
   A. Fluid resuscitation and blood pressure support while determining definitive management.
   B. Discuss risks and benefits of drainage with patient, then proceed with specialty consultation as needed for drainage (catheter drainage, emergent pericardiocentesis, surgical drainage if biopsy needed).

CORD COMPRESSION

I. **Background information**
   A. Cord compression results from thecal sac compression from neoplasms.
      1. The spinal cord distal tip usually lies at L1 with the cauda equina (lumbosacral) nerve roots just below.
      2. Most common cancers include lung, breast, multiple myeloma, lymphoma (Hodgkin's and non-Hodgkin's), and prostate.
      3. Most commonly the thoracic spine is involved, then lumbosacral spine, and finally cervical spine.

II. **Evaluation**
   A. Diagnosis is usually delayed, with most patients having back pain for 2–3 months prior to diagnosis and becoming nonambulatory by the time a diagnosis is made.
      1. Progressive back pain worsens when laying down or walking and usually precedes neurological symptoms by 1–2 months.
      2. Increasing weakness is noted with eventual loss of gait prior to paralysis.
   B. Image the entire spine as lesions may present elsewhere from where symptoms are located.
      • MRI is preferred, then CT myelography (via CSF contrast).
         a. If unable to do an MRI or CT myelography, consider CT or plain films.
            i. Can detect vertebral body damage, and in cancer patients, can assume that cord compression may be present as well, depending on history and physical examination

III. **Management**
   A. Opioid analgesia
   B. Dexamethasone: 10 mg IV ×1, then 4–6 mg IV q 6 hours while loading then switch to daily morning regimen once able
      • Switch to oral regimen as soon as possible (equivalent dosing to IV) and taper off over 1–2 weeks if definitive treatment has occurred. Utilize appropriate GI tract protection and thrush prophylaxis while on steroids.
   C. Surgical decompression evaluation by spine surgeon
      • Consider vertebroplasty/kyphoplasty (if spine unstable).
   D. Radiotherapy, unless radio-resistant neoplasm (some renal cell carcinomas and melanomas). Discuss with radiation oncologist.
   E. Chemotherapy can be considered for germ cell cancers, lymphoma, and neuroblastoma.

HYPERCALCEMIA

I. **Background information**
   A. Hypercalcemia is commonly due to hyperparathyroidism or malignancy.
   B. Usually mild with primary hyperparathyroidism but more severe (>13 mg/dL) in cancer patients.
   C. Symptom can be classified by the mnemonic "stones, bones, [abdominal] groans, and [psychiatric] moans":
      1. Stones: Kidney stones, salivary stones, renal dysfunction (polyuria), renal failure
      2. Bones: Bone pain, pathological fractures, osteomalacia
      3. Groans: GI tract (anorexia, nausea, heartburn, constipation, peptic ulcers, pancreatitis)
      4. Moans: Lethargy, fatigue, ataxia, delirium, coma (Ca++ >14 mg/dL), anxiety, depression

II. **Evaluation**
   A. Even if calcium is normal, suspicion should be high if patient's albumin is markedly decreased.
      1. The corrected calcium should be calculated or ionized calcium should be measured.
      2. Hypercalcemia of malignancy may be indirectly due to PTH-related peptide or directly due to osteolytic bone metastases.
      3. If patient does not have cancer, an intact PTH should be measured.
         a. If PTH is low, a search for malignancy or other causes should occur (such as hypercalcemia from interventions/medications like thiazide diuretics, lithium, or parenteral nutrition).

III. **Management**
   A. Increase urinary excretion.
      1. Normal saline infusion (works within hours): Up to 200–300 mL/h in patients without edema, heart failure, or renal failure and adjust for goal urine output of 100–150 mL/hr
         a. Monitor for edema or other signs of fluid overload.
      2. Loop diuretics (works within hours): Only consider in patients with heart failure or renal failure and only if needed to prevent or treat fluid overload from saline infusion
         a. Consider utilizing calcitonin instead for initial rapid reduction in calcium.
   B. Inhibit bone resorption by inhibiting osteoclasts.
      1. Calcitonin (works within hours and also promotes urinary excretion): 4 international units/kg IM/SQ q 12 h up to 6–8 international units/kg q 6 h.
         a. Nasal dosing is not helpful.
         b. Use for severe hypercalcemia for up to 48 hours.

2. Bisphosphonates (works in 1–3 days): Preferred agents and can be utilized in cancer patients with bone metastases to prevent hypercalcemia.
   a. Pamidronate: 60 mg IV (90 mg IV if Ca >13.5 mg/dL) over 2–4 hours, repeat 1–4 weeks (usually monthly for maintenance)
      i. Preferred over zoledronic acid in multiple myeloma patients due to risk of jaw osteonecrosis
   b. Zoledronic acid: 4 mg IV over 15 minutes (preferred for most cancer-related hypercalcemia) as more potent and convenient for outpatient dosing, however cost may be prohibitive
      i. Caution renal toxicity especially at higher doses than 4 mg
3. Gallium nitrate (works in 3–5 days): Consider if refractory to bisphosphonates, 200 mg/m^2/day continuous infusion for up to 5 days.
   a. Caution in renal failure patients (avoid if Cr >2.5 mg/dL).
C. Decrease GI tract absorption.
   • Glucocorticoids (takes several days to work): Prednisone 20–40 mg/day
D. Emergent hemodialysis may be required for refractory cases or patients already volume overloaded.
E. Summary
   1. If mild symptoms (such as constipation only), treat underlying cause and monitor. If moderate to severe symptoms then utilize a calcium-lowering intervention.
   2. If moderately elevated (Ca 12–14 mg/dL), but not rapidly rising can manage by treating underlying cause and reserve specific hypercalcemia treatment for patients who are symptomatic.
   3. If severely elevated (Ca >14 mg/dL), treat regardless of symptoms; utilize saline, calcitonin, and a bisphosphonate simultaneously.

INCREASED INTRACRANIAL PRESSURE

I. **Background information**
   A. Increased ICP (intracranial pressure) can occur from mass lesions, abscesses, venous outflow obstruction, and hematomas in cancer patients.
   B. Symptoms may include headache, visual changes, nausea/vomiting, and mental status changes.
   C. Signs may include:
      1. Cushing's triad (bradycardia, bradypnea, and hypertension) from brainstem compression.
      2. Unilateral or bilateral fixed/dilated pupils may be noted.
      3. Decorticate or decerebrate posturing can be observed.

II. **Evaluation**
   A. CT head, but depending on prognosis and goals of care, neurosurgical consultation should be obtained if suspected even if CT of head does not show evidence of elevated ICP

III. **Management**
   A. Definitive treatment of underlying cause (such as surgical resection).
   B. Avoid large shifts in blood pressure.
   C. Avoid cerebral perfusion pressure <60 mm Hg.
   D. Keep head of bed elevated.
   E. Hyperventilation (goal gCO_2 of 26–30 mm Hg).
   F. Medication.
      1. Mannitol: 20% 1–1.5 g/kg IV ×1, then 0.25–0.5 g/kg q 6–8 h as needed (induces an osmotic diuresis).
      2. Decrease metabolic demand (sedation with propofol, treating fevers).
      3. Dexamethasone: 10 mg IV/PO ×1, then 4–6 mg q 6 h or 8 mg q 12 h (if stable can use lower dose of 1–2 mg q 6 h) and then dose q AM once stabilized.
         a. Oral dosing starts working within 30 minutes and can be utilized unless patient unable to swallow safely.
         b. Utilize dexamethasone for tumor-related brain swelling.

SEROTONIN SYNDROME

I. **Background information**
   A. Serotonin syndrome is due to toxicity usually from 2 or more serotonergic drugs (or a high dose of 1 agent).
      1. Drugs include amphetamines (such as dextroamphetamine), levodopa, tramadol, SSRIs, SNRIs, bupropion, TCAs, dextromethorphan, MAOIs, triptans, buspirone, ergot derivatives, fentanyl, and lithium.
      2. Illicit or herbal drugs may also contribute such as cocaine, MDMA (ecstasy), St. John's wort, and LSD.

II. **Evaluation**
   A. A low index of suspicion and careful drug history is helpful.
   B. Signs include tachycardia, hypertension, fluctuating vitals, agitation, hyperthermia (temp >38°C), ocular clonus (slow horizontal motion), tremors, hyperreflexia, myoclonus, rigidity, dilated pupils, dry mouth, hyperactive bowel sounds, and diaphoresis.
   C. Develops and resolves over 24 hours, whereas the main differential of neuroleptic malignant syndrome develops and resolves over days to weeks (and has no tremor or is hyporeflexia).
   D. Labs are not required for diagnosis, but leukocytosis, renal failure, DIC, and rhabdomyolysis may develop, so basic labs and imaging can be helpful.

III. **Management**
  A. Discontinue all serotonergic medications.
  B. Supportive care: As hypotension may occur, utilize only short-acting antihypertensives (such as esmolol) if needed.
  C. Benzodiazepines as needed.
  D. Serotonin antagonist (antidote): If needed, cyproheptadine 12 mg PO ×1, then 2 mg q 2 h until sedation; may be crushed and given via NG tube.
    • Resulting hypotension should be treated with IVFs.
  E. Call American Association of Poison Control Centers for poison emergency in the United States: 1-800-222-1222.

SUPERIOR VENA CAVA SYNDROME

I. **Background information**
  A. Majority due to cancer (either direct obstruction/compression of the SVC by the cancer or thrombosis due to catheters).
  B. Because of how rapidly tumors may grow, collateral blood vessels do not have time to fully develop, but can be evident over the head, neck, and upper chest.
  C. Symptoms include head and neck tissue swelling resulting in dyspnea, stridor, and dysphagia; cerebral edema can also occur.
  D. Average lifespan if due to cancer is 6 months.
II. **Evaluation**
  A. Majority due to malignancy (and often located right side) of non-small cell lung cancer, then small cell lung cancer, then non-Hodgkin's lymphoma.
  B. Diagnosis can be confirmed by CT scan of the chest.
III. **Management**
  A. Obtain a tissue diagnosis if needed.
    • If candidate, treat underlying malignancy.
  B. Glucocorticoids if lymphoma or thymoma present or if respiratory compromise is evident.
  C. Diuretics.
  D. For rapid relief a stent should be placed, followed by anticoagulation if tolerated.
  E. Radiotherapy should be considered, may take several weeks for full benefit, but should be done emergently with a stent if respiratory compromise is evident.

TUMOR LYSIS SYNDROME

I. **Background information**
    A. Tumor lysis syndrome is due to rapid tumor cell death with resulting release of intracellular compounds.
        1. With resulting hyperkalemia and hyperphosphatemia, DNA/RNA release leads to increased uric acid, which increases risk of renal failure.
        2. Most often seen with treatment of Burkitt's lymphoma and acute lymphoblastic leukemia.
        3. Highest risk patients have some degree of baseline renal failure (creatinine >1.5 mg/dL).

II. **Evaluation**
    A. Evaluation should be proactive.
        • Monitor for symptoms of electrolyte or uric acid disturbances such as nausea, vomiting, diarrhea, lethargy, dysrhythmias, cramps, tetany, seizures, and syncope.
    B. Signs.
        1. Uric acid ≥8 mg/dL (25% increase from baseline)
        2. K ≥6 mmol/L (25% increase from baseline)
        3. Phos ≥4.5 mg/dL (25% increase from baseline)
        4. Calcium ≤7 mg/dL (25% decrease from baseline)

III. **Management**
    A. Best management is proactive and depends on prechemotherapy risk assessment by patient's oncologist.
        • Measures include IV fluid hydration (caution electrolytes in fluids), rasburicase, and allopurinol.
    B. For established tumor lysis syndrome
        1. Treat hyperphosphatemia (IVFs, hemodialysis if needed).
        2. Treat hyperkalemia (10U IV insulin/25 g glucose, sodium bicarbonate, calcium gluconate 1 g IV).
        3. Treat hypocalcemia after hyperphosphatemia treated to minimize calcium-phosphate precipitation unless tetany or dysrhythmias present (calcium gluconate 1 g IV).
        4. Rasburicase (if not used in prevention) should be initiated at 0.2 mg/kg daily for up to 5 days (follow uric acid levels as often as q 6 hours until normalized; notify lab that patient is on rasburicase for appropriate collection technique).

WITHDRAWAL SYNDROMES

TABLE 11.1 Withdrawal Syndromes

Class of Drugs	Symptoms	Signs	Management
Benzodiazepine (BDZ)	Anxiety, dysphoria, hallucinations	Tremors, fevers, seizures	Diazepam IV, then resume BDZ and taper over several months.
Corticosteroid (acute adrenal insufficiency)	Weakness, fatigue, myalgia, arthralgia, nausea, abdominal pain, confusion	Hyponatremia, hypoglycemia, vomiting, hypotension	IVF resuscitation, dexamethasone 4 mg IV ×1 (not measured in cortisol assays) or hydrocortisone 100 mg IV ×1, repeat as needed until prior steroid can be resumed, then slowly tapered if needed.
Opioid (after abrupt cessation or decrease or after receiving an antagonist)	Dysphoria, restlessness, myalgias, arthralgia, nausea, cramping, diarrhea	Rhinorrhea, lacrimation, vomiting, mydriasis, yawning, increased bowel sounds, piloerection, HTN, tachycardia	Resume opioid; avoid opioid antagonists or partial antagonists. Consider clonidine 0.1–0.3 mg PO q 1 h as needed, give benzodiazepines with clonidine if needed.
SSRI (most severe with paroxetine)	Flu-like symptoms (dizziness, nausea, fatigue, myalgias), anxiety		Cross-taper if switching from SSRI to TCA or mirtazapine over 1–2 weeks. No need to cross-taper if converting to another SSRI or venlafaxine/duloxetine. If not planning to resume SSRI then taper the prior SSRI; for withdrawal symptoms fluoxetine 10 mg daily for 1–2 weeks may help.

12 ■ FURTHER READING AND REFERENCES

CHAPTER 1: BACKGROUND

Barbera, L., Taylor, C., & Dudgeon, D. (2010). Why do patients with cancer visit the emergency department near the end of life? *Canadian Medical Association Journal, 182*(6), 563–568.

Lamba, S., Quest, T. E., & Weissman, D. E. (2011). *Emergency Department Management of Hospice Patients. Fast Facts and Concepts #246.* Retrieved 07/08/2012 from: www.eperc.mcw.edu/EPERC/FastFactsIndex/Documents/ff_246.htm.

Linzer, M., Visser, M. R., Oort, F. J., et al. (2001). Predicting and preventing physician burnout: results from the United States and the Netherlands. *The American Journal of Medicine, 111*(2), 170–175.

National Hospice and Palliative Care Organization. (2012). *NHPCO Facts and Figures: Hospice Care in America.* Alexandria, VA: National Hospice and Palliative Care Organization. Retrieved 07/08/2012 from: www.nhpco.org/files/public/statistics_research/2011_facts_figures.pdf.

CHAPTER 2: COMMUNICATION

Ambuel, B., & Weissman, D. E. (2005). *Moderating an End-of-Life Family Conference, 2nd ed. Fast Facts and Concepts #16.* Retrieved 07/08/2012 from: www.eperc.mcw.edu/fastfact/ff_016.htm.

Back, A., Arnold, R., & Tulsky, J. (2009). *Mastering Communication with Seriously Ill Patients: Balancing Honesty with Empathy and Hope.* New York: Cambridge University Press.

Chaitin, E., & Rosielle, D. (2009). *Responding to Requests for Non-Disclosure of Medical Information. Fast Facts and Concepts #219.* Retrieved 07/08/2012 from: www.eperc.mcw.edu/EPERC/FastFactsIndex/ff_219.htm

Kendall, A., & Arnold, R. (2007). *Conflict Resolution I: Careful Communication. Fast Facts and Concepts #183.* Retrieved 07/08/2012 from: www.eperc.mcw.edu/fastfact/ff_183.htm.

Kendall, A., & Arnold, R. (2007). *Conflict Resolution II: Principled Negotiation. Fast Facts and Concepts #184.* Retrieved 07/08/2012 from: www.eperc.mcw.edu/fastfact/ff_184.htm.

Platt, F. W., Gaspar, D. L., & Coulehan, J. L. (2001). "Tell me about yourself": The patient-centered interview. *Annals of Internal Medicine, 134*(11), 1079–1085.

Quill, T. E., Arnold, R. M., & Platt, F. (2001). "I wish things were different": expressing wishes in response to loss, futility, and unrealistic hopes. *Annals of Internal Medicine, 135*(7), 551–555.

Weissman, D. E., Quill, T. E., & Arnold, R. M. (2010). *Helping Surrogates Make Decisions. Fast Facts and Concepts #226.* Retrieved 07/08/2012 from: www.eperc.mcw.edu/fastfact/ff_226.htm.

CHAPTER 3: ETHICAL DECISION MAKING

Jonsen, A. R., Siegler, M., & Winslade, W. J. (2002). *Clinical Ethics: A Practical Approach to Ethical Decisions in Clinical Medicine*, 5th ed. New York: McGraw-Hill.

Junkerman, C., & Schiedermayer, D. (1998). *Practical Ethics for Students, Interns, and Residents: A Short Reference Manual*, 2nd ed. Frederick, MD: University Publishing Group, Inc.

Macauley, R. (2011). Patients who make "wrong" choices. *Journal of Palliative Medicine, 14*(1), 13–16.

Tarzian, A. (chair). (2011). *Core Competencies for Healthcare Ethics Consultation*, 2nd ed. Glenview, IL: American Society for Bioethics and Humanities.

Watkins, L. T., Sacajiu, G., & Karasz, A. (2007). The role of the bioethicist in family meetings about end of life care. *Social Science & Medicine, 65*(11), 2328–2341.

Wijdicks, E. F., Varelas, P. N., Gronseth, G. S., & Greer, D. M. (2010). Evidence-based guideline update: determining brain death in adults: report of the Quality Standards Subcommittee of the American Academy of Neurology. *Neurology, 74*(23), 1911–1918.

CHAPTER 4: PROGNOSTICATION

Beddhu, S., Bruns, F. J., Saul, M., Seddon, P., & Zeidel, M. L. (2000). A simple comorbidity scale predicts clinical outcomes and costs in dialysis patients. *American Journal of Medicine, 108*(8), 609–613.

Carson, S. S., Garrett, J., Hanson, L. C., et al. (2008). A prognostic model for one-year mortality in patients requiring prolonged mechanical ventilation. *Critical Care Medicine, 36*(7), 2061–2069.

Cohen, L. M., Ruthazer, R., Moss, A. H., & Germain, M. J. (2010). Predicting six-month mortality for patients who are on maintenance hemodialysis. *Clinical Journal of the American Society of Nephrology, 5*(1), 72–79.

Durand, F., & Valla, D. (2005). Assessment of the prognosis of cirrhosis: Child-Pugh versus MELD. *Journal of Hepatology, 42*(Suppl 1), S100–S107.

Howlader, N., Noone, A. M., Krapcho, M., et al. (eds). (2012). *SEER Cancer Statistics Review, 1975–2009 (Vintage 2009 Populations)*. Bethesda, MD: National Cancer Institute. Retrieved 7/10/2012 from: http://seer.cancer.gov/csr/1975_2009_pops09/, based on November 2011 SEER data submission, posted to the SEER web site, April 2012.

Lin, E., & Lozano, R. (2010). *Cancer-Matrix Manual*, 5th ed. Madison, WI: Advanced Medical Publishing, Inc.

Maltoni, M., Nanni, O., Pirovano, M., et al. (1999). Successful validation of the palliative prognostic score in terminally ill cancer patients. *Journal of Pain and Symptom Management, 17*(4), 240–247.

Morita, T., Tsunoda, J., Inoue, S., & Chihara, S. (1999). The Palliative Prognostic Index: a scoring system for survival prediction of terminally ill cancer patients. *Supportive Care in Cancer, 7*(3), 128–133.

Puhan, M. A., Garcia-Aymerich, J., Frey, M., et al. (2009). Expansion of the prognostic assessment of patients with chronic obstructive pulmonary disease: the updated BODE index and the ADO index. *Lancet, 374*(9691), 704–711.

Tian, J., Kaufman, D. A., Zarich, S., et al. (2010). Outcomes of critically ill patients who received cardiopulmonary resuscitation. *American Journal of Respiratory and Critical Care Medicine, 182*(4), 501–506.

U.S. Cancer Statistics Working Group. (2012). United States Cancer Statistics: 1999–2008 Incidence and Mortality Web-based Report. Atlanta, GA: U.S. Department of Health and Human Services, Centers for Disease Control and Prevention and National Cancer Institute. Retrieved 7/10/2012 from: www.cdc.gov/uscs

Walter, L. C., Brand, R. J., Counsell, S. R., et al. (2001). Development and validation of a prognostic index for 1–year mortality in older adults after hospitalization. *Journal of the American Medical Association, 285*(23), 2987–2994.

Warm, E. J. (2005). *Prognostication, 2nd ed. Fast Facts and Concepts #30.* Retrieved 07/08/2012 from: www.eperc.mcw.edu/fastfact/ff_030.htm.

Weissman, D. E. (2005). *Determining Prognosis in Advanced Cancer, 2nd ed. Fast Facts and Concepts #13.* Retrieved 07/08/2012 from: www.eperc.mcw.edu/fastfact/ff_013.htm.

CHAPTER 5: CULTURAL AND RELIGIOUS CONCERNS

Doka, K. J. (2011). Religion and spirituality: assessment and intervention. *Journal of Social Work in End-of-Life & Palliative Care 7*, 99–109.

LaRocca-Pitts, M. (2009). In FACT, chaplains have a spiritual assessment tool. *American Journal of Pastoral Care and Health, 3*(2), 8–15.

Lipson, J. G., Dibble, S. L., & Minarik, P. A. (Eds.). (2003). *Culture & Nursing Care: A Pocket Guide.* San Francisco, CA: UCSF Nursing Press.

CHAPTER 6 : GASTROINTESTINAL AND GENITOURINARY

6.1: ANOREXIA-CACHEXIA SYNDROME

Gordon, J. N., Trebble, T. M., Ellis, R. D., Duncan, H. D., Johns, T., & Goggin, P. M. (2005). Thalidomide in the treatment of cancer cachexia: a randomized placebo controlled trial. *Gut, 54*(4), 540–545.

Jatoi, A., Windschitl, H. E., Loprinzi, C. L., et al. (2002). Dronabinol versus megestrol acetate versus combination therapy for cancer-associated anorexia: A North Central Cancer Treatment Group study. *Journal of Clinical Oncology, 20*(2), 567–573.

Kotler, D. (2000). Cachexia. *Annals of Internal Medicine, 133*(8), 622–634.

Lissoni, P., Paolorossi, F., Ardizzoia, A., et al. (1997). A randomized study of chemotherapy with cisplatin plus etoposide versus chemoendocrine therapy with cisplatin, etoposide and the pineal hormone melatonin as a first-line treatment of advanced non-small cell lung cancer patients in a poor clinical state. *Journal of Pineal Research, 23*(1), 15–19.

Loprinzi, C. L., Kugler, J. W., Sloan, J. A., et al. (1999). Randomized comparison of megestrol acetate versus dexamethasone versus fluoxymesterone

for the treatment of cancer anorexia/cachexia. *Journal of Clinical Oncology, 17*(10), 3299–3306.

Moertel, C. G., Kvols, L. K., & Rubin, J. (1991). A study of cyproheptadine in the treatment of metastatic carcinoid tumor and the malignant carcinoid syndrome. *Cancer, 67*(1), 33–36.

Yavuzsen, T., Davis, M. P., Walsh, D., LeGrand, S., & Lagman, R. (2005). Systematic review of the treatment of cancer-associated anorexia and weight loss. *Journal of Clinical Oncology, 23*(33), 8500–8511.

6.2: ASCITES, MALIGNANCY-RELATED

Adam, R. A., & Adam, Y. G. (2004). Malignant ascites: past, present, and future. *Journal of the American College of Surgeons, 198*(6), 999–1011.

Becker, G., Galandi, D., & Blum H. E. (2006). Malignant ascites: systematic review and guideline for treatment. *European Journal of Cancer, 42*(5), 589–597.

Cairns, W., & Malone, R. (1999). Octreotide as an agent for the relief of malignant ascites in palliative care patients. *Palliative Medicine, 13*(5), 429–430.

Kobold, S., Hegewisch-Becker, S., Oechsle, K., Jordan, K., Bokemeyer, C., & Atanackovic, D. (2009). Intraperitoneal VEGF inhibition using bevacizumab: a potential approach for the symptomatic treatment of malignant ascites? *Oncologist, 14*(12), 1242–1251.

Singh, V., Dheerendra, P. C., Singh, B., et al. (2008). Midodrine versus albumin in the prevention of paracentesis-induced circulatory dysfunction in cirrhotics: a randomized pilot study. *American Journal of Gastroenterology, 103*(6), 1399–1405.

6.3: URINARY SYMPTOMS

Chapple, C., Khullar, V., Gabriel, Z., & Dooley, J. A. (2005). The effects of antimuscarinic treatments in overactive bladder: a systematic review and meta-analysis. *European Urology, 48*(1), 5–26.

Fink, H. A., Taylor, B. C., Tacklind, J. W., Rutks, I. R., & Wilt, T. J. (2008). Treatment interventions in nursing home residents with urinary incontinence: a systematic review of randomized trials. *Mayo Clinic Proceedings, 83*(12), 1332–1343.

van Ophoven, A., & Hertle, L. (2005). Long-term results of amitriptyline treatment for interstitial cystitis. *The Journal of Urology, 174*(5), 1837–1840.

Verhamme, K. M., Sturkenboom, M. C., Stricker, B. H., & Bosch, R. (2008). Drug-induced urinary retention: incidence, management, and prevention. *Drug Safety, 31*(5), 373–388.

Zinner, N., Gittelman, M., Harris, R., et al. (2004). Trospium chloride improves overactive bladder symptoms: a multicenter phase III trial. *The Journal of Urology, 171*(6 Pt 1), 2311–2315.

6.4: ABDOMINAL BLOATING AND GAS

Ganiats, T. G., Norcross, W. A., Halverson, A. L., Burford, P. A., & Palinkas, L. A. (1994). Does Beano prevent gas? A double-blind crossover study of oral alpha-galactosidase to treat dietary oligosaccharide intolerance. *The Journal of Family Practice, 39*(5), 441–445.

Jain, N. K., Patel, V. P., & Pitchumoni, C. S. (1986). Activated charcoal, simethicone, and intestinal gas: a double-blind study. *Annals of Internal Medicine, 105*(1), 61–62.

6.5: CONSTIPATION AND BOWEL OBSTRUCTION

Bruera, E. & Fadul, N. (2009). Constipation. In Bruera, E., Higginson, I. J., Ripamonti, C., & von Gunten, C. (Eds.), *Textbook of Palliative Medicine* (pp. 554–560). London: Hodder Arnold.

Caroline, N. & Waller, A. (1996). Constipation. In Waller, A., & Caroline, N. L., *Handbook of Palliative Care in Cancer* (pp. 169–176). Newton, MA: Butterworth- Heinemann.

Jatoi, A., Podratz, K. C., Gill, P., & Hartmann, L. C. (2004). Pathophysiology and palliation of inoperable bowel obstruction in patients with ovarian cancer. *The Journal of Supportive Oncology, 2*(4), 323–334.

Lembo, A., & Camilleri, M. Chronic constipation. *The New England Journal of Medicine, 349*(14), 1360–1368.

Meissner, W., Schmidt, U., Hartmann, M., Kath, R., & Reinhart, K. (2000). Oral naloxone reverses opioid-associated constipation. *Pain, 84*(1), 105–109.

Ripamonti, C., & Mercadante S. (2004). How to use octreotide for malignant bowel obstruction. *Journal of Supportive Oncology, 2*, 357–364.

Ripamonti, C., Mercadante, S., Groff, L., et al. (2000). Role of octreotide, scopolamine butylbromide, and hydration in symptom control of patients with inoperable bowel obstruction and nasogastric tubes: a prospective, random-ized trial. *Journal of Pain and Symptom Management,* 19, 23–34.

6.6: DIARRHEA

Fine, K. D., & Schiller, L. R. (1999). AGA medical position statement: guide-lines for the evaluation of chronic diarrhea. *Gastroenterology, 116*(6), 1461–1463.

Yeoh, E. K., Horowitz, M., Russo, A., Muecke, T., Robb, T., & Chatterton, B. E. (1993). Gastrointestinal function in chronic radiation enteritis—effects of loperamide-N-oxide. *Gut, 34*(4), 476–482.

6.7: DYSPEPSIA AND GASTROESOPHAGEAL REFLUX DISEASE (GERD)

Jackson, J. L., O'Malley, P. G., Tomkins, G., Balden, E., Santoro, J., & Kroenke, K. (2000). Treatment of functional gastrointestinal disorders with antidepressant medications: a meta-analysis. *American Journal of Medicine, 108*(1), 65–72.

Kahrilas, P. J., Shaheen, N. J., & Vaezi, M. F. (2008). American Gastroenterological Association Institute technical review on the management of gastroesophageal reflux disease. *Gastroenterology, 135*(4), 1392–1413.

Talley, N. J. (2005). American Gastroenterological Association medi-cal position statement: evaluation of dyspepsia. *Gastroenterology, 129*(5), 1753–1755.

6.8: OROPHARYNX: DYSPHAGIA, MUCOSITIS, XEROSTOMIA, HALITOSIS

Fusco, F. (2009). Mouth care. In Bruera, E., Higginson, I. J., Ripamonti, C., & von Gunten, C. (Eds.), *Textbook of Palliative Medicine* (pp. 773–779). London: Hodder Arnold.

Porter, S. R., & Scully, C. (2006). Oral malodour (halitosis). *BMJ, 333*(7569), 632–635.

Waller, A., & Caroline, N. L. (1996). Oral complications and mouth care. In Waller, A., & Caroline, N. L. *Handbook of Palliative Care in Cancer* (pp. 113–122). Boston: Butterworth-Heinemann.

Wrede-Seaman, L. (2009). Candidiasis. In Wrede-Seaman, L., *Symptom Management Algorithms: A Handbook for Palliative Care* (3rd ed., pp. 37–38). Yakima: Intellicard, Inc.

6.9: NAUSEA AND VOMITING

Bruera, E., & Neumann, C. M. (1998). Management of specific symptom complexes in patients receiving palliative care. *Canadian Medical Association Journal, 158*(13), 1717–1726.

Flake, Z. A., Scalley, R. D., & Bailey, A. G. (2004). Practical selection of antiemetics. *American Family Physician, 69*(5), 1169–1174.

Jackson, W. C., & Tavernier, L. (2003). Olanzapine for intractable nausea in palliative care patients. *Journal of Palliative Medicine, 6*(2), 251–255.

Keeley, P. W. (2009). Nausea and vomiting in people with cancer and other chronic diseases. *Clinical Evidence (online)*, Jan. 13.

Wood, G. J., Shega, J. W., Lynch, B., & Von Roenn, J. H. (2007). Management of intractable nausea and vomiting in patients at the end of life: "I was feeling nauseous all of the time…nothing was working." *JAMA, 298*(10), 1196–1207.

CHAPTER 7: NEUROPSYCHIATRIC

7.1: ANXIETY

Kinzbrunner, B. M., & Policzer, J. S. (Eds.) (2011). Delirium, depression, and anxiety. In Kinzbrunner, B. M., & Policzer, J. S. (Eds.), *End-of-Life Care: A Practical Guide* (2nd ed., pp. 276–279). New York: McGraw-Hill.

Quill, T. E. (2007). Depression and anxiety. In Quill, T. E., *Primer of Palliative Care* (4th ed., pp. 61–66). Glenview, IL: AAHPM.

Waller, A., & Caroline, N. L. (1996). Anxiety. In Waller, A., & Caroline, N. L. *Handbook of Palliative Care in Cancer* (pp. 295–299). Boston: Butterworth-Heinemann.

Wrede-Seaman, L. (2009). Anxiety assessment. In Wrede-Seaman, L., *Symptom Management Algorithms: A Handbook for Palliative Care* (3rd ed., pp. 20–21). Yakima: Intellicard.

7.2: DELIRIUM

Inouye, S. K., Bogardus, S. T., Jr., Charpentier, P. A., et al. (1999). A multicomponent intervention to prevent delirium in hospitalized older patients. *New England Journal of Medicine, 340*(1999), 669–676.

Inouye, S. K., van Dyck, C. H., Alessi, C. A., Balkin, S., Siegal, A. P., & Horwitz, R. I. (1990). Clarifying confusion: the confusion assessment method. A new method for detection of delirium. *Annals of Internal Medicine, 113*(12), 941–948.

Kinzbrunner, B. M., & Policzer, J. S. (Eds.) (2011). Delirium, depression, and anxiety. In Kinzbrunner, B. M., & Policzer, J. S. (Eds.), *End-of-Life Care: A Practical Guide* (2nd ed., pp. 263–269). New York: McGraw-Hill.

Rousseau, P. (2004). Palliative sedation in the management of refractory symptoms. *Journal of Supportive Oncology, 2*(2), 181–186.

Twycross, R., & Wilcock, A. (Eds.) (2008). Phenobarbital. In Twycross, R., & Wilcock, A. (Eds.), *Hospice and Palliative Care Formulary USA* (2nd ed., pp. 213–216). United Kingdom: Palliativedrugs.com Ltd.

Twycross, R., & Wilcock, A. (Eds.) (2008). Propofol. In Twycross, R., & Wilcock, A. (Eds.), *Hospice and Palliative Care Formulary USA* (2nd ed., pp. 462–465). United Kingdom: Palliativedrugs.com Ltd.

7.3: GRIEF AND BEREAVEMENT

Bruce, C. A. (2002). The grief process for patient, family, and physician. *Journal of the American Osteopathic Association, 102*(9 Suppl 3), S28–S32.

National Cancer Institute. Grief, Bereavement, and Coping With Loss (PDQ). Bethesda, MD: National Cancer Institute. Date last modified August 31, 2010. Retrieved 4/5/2011 from: http://cancer.gov/cancertopics/pdq/supportivecare/bereavement/HealthProfessional.

Shanafelt, T., Adjei, A., & Meyskens, F. L. (2003). When your favorite patient relapses: physician grief and well-being in the practice of oncology. *Journal of Clinical Oncology, 21*(13), 2616–2619.

Worden, J. W. (2009). Grief counseling: facilitating uncomplicated grief. In Worden, J. W., *Grief Counseling and Grief Therapy: A Handbook for the Mental Health Practitioner* (4th ed., pp. 31, 83). New York: Springer Publishing.

7.4: DEPRESSION

Block, S. D. (2000). Assessing and managing depression in the terminally ill patient. *Annals of Internal Medicine, 132*(3), 209–218.

Nierenberg, A. A., Fava, M., Trivedi, M. H., et al. (2006). A comparison of lithium and T3 augmentation following two failed medication treatments for depression: a STAR*D report. *The American Journal of Psychiatry, 163*(9), 1519–1530.

Price, C. S., & Taylor F. B. (2005). A retrospective chart review of the effects of modafinil on depression as monotherapy and as adjunctive therapy. *Depression and Anxiety, 21*(4), 149–153.

Rozans, M., Dreisbach, A., Lertora J. J., & Kahn, M. J. (2002). Palliative uses of methylphenidate in patients with cancer: a review. *Journal of Clinical Oncology, 20*(1), 335–339.

Zarate, C. A. Jr., Singh, J. B., Carlson, P. J., et al. (2006). A randomized trial of an N-methyl-D-aspartate antagonist in treatment-resistant major depression. *Archives of General Psychiatry, 63*(8), 856–864.

7.5: FATIGUE

Boohene, J. A., & Bruera, E. (2009). Treatment of fatigue in palliative care. In Bruera, E., Higginson, I. J., Ripamonti, C., & von Gunten, C. (Eds.), *Textbook of Palliative Medicine* (pp. 639–649). London: Hodder Arnold.

Minton, O., Richardson, A., Sharpe, M., Hotopf, M., & Stone, P. (2008). A systematic review and meta-analysis of the pharmacological treatment of cancer-related fatigue. *Journal of the National Cancer Institute, 100*(16), 1155–1166.

Renier-Berg, D. M. (2003). General issues: fatigue, dyspnea, and constipation. In Forman, W. B., Kitzes, J. A., Anderson, R. P., & Kopchak Sheehan, D. (Eds.), *Hospice and Palliative Care: Concepts and Practice* (2nd ed., pp. 129–142). Sudbury, MA: Jones and Bartlett.

7.6: INSOMNIA

Krystal, A. D. (2009). A compendium of placebo-controlled trials of the risks/benefits of pharmacological treatments for insomnia: the empirical basis for U.S. clinical practice. *Sleep Medicine Reviews, 13*(4), 265–274.

Miller, M., & Arnold, R. (2004). *Insomnia: Pharmacological Therapies. Fast Facts and Concepts #105.* Retrieved from: www.eperc.mcw.edu/fastfact/ff_105.htm.

CHAPTER 8: PAIN

Alford, D. P., Liebschutz, J., Chen, I. A., et al. (2008). Update in pain medicine. *Journal of General Internal Medicine, 23*(6), 841–845.

Berde, C. B., & Sethna, N. F. (2002). Analgesics for the treatment of pain in children. *The New England Journal of Medicine, 347*(14), 1094–1103.

Brooks, P. M, & Day, R. O. (1991). Nonsteroidal anti-inflammatory drugs—differences and similarities. *New England Journal of Medicine, 324*(24), 1716–1725.

Gazelle, G., & Fine, P. G. (2006). *Methadone for the Treatment of Pain, 2nd ed. Fast Facts and Concepts #75.* Retrieved from: www.eperc.mcw.edu/fastfact/ff_075.htm.

Kerr, C., Holahan, T., & Milch, R. (2011). The use of ketamine in severe cases of refractory pain syndromes in the palliative care setting: a case series. *Journal of Palliative Medicine, 14*(9), 1074–1077.

Kishore, A., King, L., & Weissman, D. E. (2005). *Gabapentin for Neuropathic Pain, 2nd ed. Fast Facts and Concepts #49.* Retrieved 7/08/2012 from: www.eperc.mcw.edu/fastfact/ff_049.htm.

McPherson, M. L. (2010). *Demystifying Opioid Conversion Calculations: A Guide for Effective Dosing.* Bethesda, MD: American Society of Health-System Pharmacists.

Moryl, N., Coyle, N., & Foley, K. M. (2008). Managing an acute pain crisis in a patient with advanced cancer: "this is as much of a crisis as a code." *Journal of the American Medical Association, 299*(12), 1457–1467.

Shaiova, L., Berger, A., Blinderman, C. D., et al. (2008). Consensus guideline on parenteral methadone use in pain and palliative care. *Palliative and Supportive Care, 6*(2), 165–176.

Von Gunten, C. F. (2007). *Methadone: Starting Dosing Information, 2nd ed. Fast Facts and Concepts #86.* Retrieved 7/08/2012 from: www.eperc.mcw.edu/fastfact/ff_086.htm.

CHAPTER 9: RESPIRATORY

9.1: CHRONIC COUGH

Doona, M., & Walsh, D. (1998). Benzonatate for opioid-resistant cough in advanced cancer. *Palliative Medicine, 12*(1), 55–58.

Morice, A. H., Menon, M. S., Mulrennan, S. A., et al. (2007). Opiate therapy in chronic cough. *American Journal of Respiratory and Critical Care Medicine, 175*(4), 312–315.

9.2: DYSPNEA

Kamal, A. H., et al. (2011). Dyspnea review for the palliative care professional: assessment, burdens, and etiologies. *Journal of Palliative Medicine, 14*(10), 1167–1172.

Kamal, A. H., et al. (2012). "Dyspnea review for the palliative care professional: treatment goals and therapeutic options." *Journal of Palliative Medicine, 15*(1), 106–114.

9.3: HICCUPS
Kinzbrunner, B. M., & Wright, J. B. (2011). Other common symptoms near the end of life. In Kinzbrunner, B. M., & Policzer, J. S. (Eds.), *End-of-Life Care: A Practical Guide* (2nd ed., pp. 337–338). New York: McGraw-Hill.

9.4: ORAL SECRETIONS
Thomas, J. R., & von Gunten, C. F. (2003). Management of dyspnea. *The Journal of Supportive Oncology, 1*(1),23–32.

CHAPTER 10: SKIN

10.1: MALODOROUS FUNGATING WOUNDS
da Costa Santos, C. M., de Mattos Pimenta, C. A., & Nobre, M. R. (2010). A systematic review of topical treatments to control the odor of malignant fungating wounds *Journal of Pain and Symptom Management, 39*(6), 1065–1076.

Ferris, F., & von Gunten, C. F. (2005). *Malignant Wounds, 2nd ed, Fast Facts and Concepts #46.* Retrieved 7/08/2012 from: www.eperc.mcw.edu/fastfact/ff_046.htm.

Patel, B., & Cox-Hayley, D. (2009). *Managing Wound Odor. Fast Facts and Concepts #218.* Retrieved 7/08/2012 from: www.eperc.mcw.edu/fastfact/ff_218.htm.

10.2: PRESSURE ULCERS
Ferris, F., & von Gunten, C. F. (2005). *Pressure Ulcer Management: Prevention (Part 1), 2nd ed. Fast Facts and Concepts #40.* Retrieved 7/08/2012 from: www.eperc.mcw.edu/fastfact/ff_040.htm.

Froiland, K. G. (2009). Pressure ulcers/wounds. In Bruera, E., Higginson, I. J., Ripamonti, C., & von Gunten, C. (Eds.), *Textbook of Palliative Medicine,* (pp. 768–772). London: Hodder Arnold.

von Gunten, C. F., & Ferris, F. (2005). *Pressure Ulcers: Debridement & Dressings (Part 2), 2nd ed. Fast Facts and Concepts #41.* Retrieved 7/08/2012 from: www.eperc.mcw.edu/fastfact/ff_041.htm.

10.3: PRURITUS
Lidstone, V., & Thorns, A. (2009). Pruritus. In Bruera, E., Higginson, I. J., Ripamonti, C., & von Gunten, C. (Eds.), *Textbook of Palliative Medicine,* (pp. 750–760). London: Hodder Arnold.

Patel, T., & Yosipovitch, G. (2010). Therapy of pruritus. *Expert Opinion on Pharmacotherapy, 11*(10), 1673–1682.

CHAPTER 11: EMERGENCIES

Warner, C. H., Bobo, W., Warner, C., Reid, S., & Rachal, J. (2006). Antidepressant discontinuation syndrome. *American Family Physician, 74*(3), 449–456.

INDEX

Note: Italicized pages indicate figures; tables are noted with t.

A

Abdominal bloating and gas, background information, evaluation, management, 55

Abstral, prescribing tips, 96

Acetaminophen, for pain management, 89, 90t

Acetylsalicylic acid, for pain management, 90t

Actiq, 95

Actively dying, 123–124
  background information, 123
  evaluation, stages of, 123–124
  management, 124

Acute bleeding, 124–125
  background information, 124–125
  evaluation and management, 125

Acyclovir, for HSV, 64

Addiction, to opioids, 101

ADO Index, 36t–37t

Adolescents, hydromorphone dosages for, 94

Adult failure to thrive, hospice criteria, 32t

Adults
  documenting pain in, 88
  fentanyl IV dosages, 97
  grief management for, 78t
  hydromorphone dosages, 94
  morphine dosages, 94
  opioid-naive, methadone dosages, 98–99
  oxycodone dosages, 95
  tramadol dosages, 100

Advance care planning documentation, 27

Advance directives, 19, 27

African Americans, views of suffering and dying by, 39t

Africans, views of suffering and dying by, 39t

AIDET mnemonic, 19

AIDS. See HIV/AIDS

Alprazolam, for anxiety, 71t

American Academy of Neurology, brain death criteria, 29

American Association of Poison Control Centers, 131

American Massage Therapy Association, 108

American Music Therapy Association, 108

American Society for Bioethics and Humanities, 24

Aminocaproic acid, for acute bleeding, 125

Amitriptyline
  for anxiety, 71t
  for depression, 82t
  for neuropathic pain, 103

Anabolic agents, for anorexia-cachexia syndrome, 50t

Analgesics, non-opioid, 90t–92t

Anaphylaxis, background information, evaluation, management, 126

Anesthetics, for neuropathic pain, 105

Anger, responding to, 17

Anglicans (Church of England), views of suffering and dying by, 41t

Anorexia-cachexia syndrome, 49–51
  background information, 49–50
  evaluation and management, 50
  treating, medications for, 50t–51t

Anorexia nervosa, 69*t*
Antibiotics, for dyspnea, 110
Anticatabolic-anticytokine agents, for anorexia-cachexia syndrome, 51*t*
Anticholinergics
    for bowel obstruction, 59*t*
    for nausea management, 67*t*
Anticipatory (or preparatory) grief, 76
Anticonvulsant medications, for neuropathic pain, 104
Antidepressants
    for anorexia-cachexia syndrome, 51*t*
    for insomnia, 86*t*
    for neuropathic pain, 103–104
Antiemetics, for bowel obstruction, 59*t*
Antifibrinolytic agents, for acute bleeding, 125
Antihistamines
    for nausea management, 67*t*
    for pruritus, 119
    for urinary retention or overflow incontinence, 55
Antipsychotics, for urinary retention or overflow incontinence, 55
Antispasmodics, for pain management
Antivert, for nausea management, 67*t*
Anxiety
    background information, 69
    cognitive interventions, 70
    disease- and medication-related causes of, 70*t*
    evaluation, 69
    fears/potential diagnosis, 69*t*
    medical interventions, 70
    pharmacological interventions for, 71*t*–72*t*
Anzemet, for nausea management, 67*t*
Apnea test, 29–30

Appetite stimulants, 51*t*
Aprepitant, for nausea management, 68*t*
Arabs, views of suffering and dying by, 39*t*
Aromatherapy, 70
Artificial nutrition and hydration, 51*t*. *See also* Shared decision making
ASBH. *See* American Society for Bioethics and Humanities
Ascites, malignancy-related, 52–53
    background and evaluation, 52
    management, 52–53
"Ask-tell-ask," 19
Aspirin
    for pain management, 90*t*
    for polycythemia vera, 120
Atarax/Vistaril, for nausea management, 67*t*
Atropine, for oral secretions, 113
Autonomy
    clinical ethics, 23
    enhanced, 18
    informed consent and, 28
Avinza, prescribing tips, 94

B
Baclofen
    for hiccups, 112
    for pain management, 104
Bad news, serious findings, poor prognosis, or nearing end-of-life, 16–18
Beano, for abdominal bloating and gas, 55
Belladonna, for bladder or ureteral spasms, 54–55
Benadryl, for nausea management, 67*t*
Beneficence, clinical ethics, 23
Benzodiazepines
    for anxiety, 71*t*
    for dyspnea, 110
    for insomnia, 85*t*
    for nausea management, 68*t*

for terminal extubation
protocols, 114
withdrawal syndromes, 133*t*
Bereavement. *See* Grief and
bereavement
"Best interest" standard, 28
Bethanechol
for constipation, 58*t*
for urinary retention or overflow
incontinence, 55
Biofeedback, for pain
management, 108
Biofeedback Certification Institute
of America, 108
Bisacodyl, for constipation, 57*t*
Bismuth subsalicylate, for
diarrhea, 61
Bisphosphonates
for hypercalcemia, 129
pain management and, 103
Bladder spasms, management,
54–55
Bleeding, acute, 124–125
Bone pain, management, 107
Bowel obstruction
background information and
evaluation, 56
management of, 58
medications, 59*t*
Brain death, diagnosis, 29
Brain stem reflexes, absence
of, 29
Breakthrough pain
opioids for, 95
types of, 89
Breathing exercises,
for anxiety, 70
Bronchodilators, for dyspnea, 110
Budd-Chiari syndrome, 52
Buddhists, views of suffering and
dying by, 41*t*
Buprenorphine, equianalgesic &
pharmacokinetic
table, 162*t*
Buproprion, for depression, 81*t*
Burnout/burnout-reduction
techniques, 12

Buspirone
for anxiety, 72*t*
for depression, 82*t*

C
Cachexia. *See* Anorexia-cachexia
syndrome
Calamine lotion, for pruritus, 119
Calcitonin, 103
Cancer
ED visit diagnosis
reasons, 6*t*
hospice criteria, 32*t*
prognosis guidelines, 35
ten deadliest, of both sexes from
all ethnicities, 36*t*
Candidiasis, management, 64
Cannabinoids
for anorexia-cachexia
syndrome, 51*t*
for nausea management, 68*t*
for neuropathic pain, 105
Capsaicin cream
for neuropathic pain, 105
for neuropathic pruritus, 120
for uremia, 120
Carbamazepine, for neuropathic
pain, 104
Cardiac tamponade, background
information, evaluation,
management, 126
Carisoprodol, for pain
management, 104
Catholics, views of suffering and
dying by, 41*t*
Cautery, for bleeding from
malodorous fungating
wounds, 116
Celecoxib, for pain
management, 92*t*
Charlson comorbidity
scale, 38
Chemoreceptor trigger
zone, 66
Chemotherapy, for ascites, 53
Cheyne-Stokes respirations, 123
Child-Pugh class, 37, 38*t*

Children
documenting pain in, 88–89
fentanyl IV dosages, 97
grief in, 76
hydromorphone dosages, 94
managing grief for different
groups, 78t–79t
methadone dosages, 98
morphine dosages, 94
oxycodone dosages, 95
tramadol dosages, 100
views of death, 7, 8t
Chinese, views of suffering and
dying by, 39t
Chlorpromazine
for anxiety, 71t
for delirium, 74t
for hiccups, 112
for nausea management, 67t
Cholestasis, 120
Cholestyramine, 120
for hematologic tumors, 119
for radiation-induced
diarrhea, 61
for uremia, 119
Choline magnesium trisalicylate, for
pain management, 90t
Christian Science, views of
suffering and dying in, 42t
"Chunk and check," 19
Cimetidine
for polycythemia vera, 120
for tumor-related pruritus, 119
Cirrhosis, pain management
and, 107
Citalopram
for anxiety, 71t
for depression, 81t
Clinical ethics, 23
Clomipramine, for anxiety, 71t
Clonazepam
for anxiety, 71t
for neuropathic pain, 104
Clonidine
for diarrhea, 61
for pain management, 104
Clotrimazole, for candidiasis, 64

Codeine
for chronic cough, 109
equianalgesic & pharmacokinetic
table, 162t
Cognitive behavioral therapy, for
anxiety, 70
Coma, hospice criteria, 34t
Comatose, brain death
diagnosis, 29
Communication, 11–21
bad news, 16–18
family, 18–21
palliative care teams, 11–12
patient, 13–16
Compazine, for nausea
management, 67t
Complicated grief
risk factors, 77–78
types, 77
Condolence card, writing, 79
Conflicts
ethics consultation and, 24
family, 21
palliative care team, 12
Confusion Assessment Method
(CAM), delirium
screening, 73t
Constipation, 56–58
background information,
evaluation,
management, 56
medications for, 57t–58t
opioids and, 100
Cord compression, background
information, evaluation,
management, 127
Corticosteroids
for anorexia-cachexia
syndrome, 51t
for dyspnea, 110
for pain management, 103
withdrawal syndromes, 133t
Cough, chronic, background
information, evaluation,
management, 109
CTZ. See Chemoreceptor
trigger zone

Cultural identity, views of suffering and dying related to, 39t–40t
Cushing's triad, 129
Cyclobenzaprine, for pain management, 104
Cyproheptadine, for anorexia-cachexia syndrome, 51t

D

Death and dying, 29–30
　Apnea test, 29–30
　brain death diagnosis, 29
　children's views of, 7, 8t
　confirmatory tests, 30
　defined, 29
　ethnic views of, 39t–40t
　fear of, 13
　religious views of, 41t–43t
"Death rattle," 112, 123, 124
Decisional capacity assessment, 27
Decision making, 13. *See also*
　　Ethical decision making
　shared, 27–28
Deep breathing, for pain management, 108
Delirium, 72–75
　background information, 72
　common etiologies, 73t
　evaluation, 73
　nonpharmacologic intervention for, 73t
　opioids and, 100
　pharmacologic intervention for, 74t
　refractory symptoms of, sedation, 75, 75t
　risk factors for, 72t
　screening, Confusion Assessment Method for, 73t
DELIRIUM mnemonic, 73t
Dementia
　hospice criteria, 32t
　prognosis guidelines for, 38
Depakote, for neuropathic pain, 105

Depression, 79–83
　background information, 79
　interview, 80
　pharmacotherapy for, 80t–82t
　psychiatry referral triggers, 83
　risk factors for, 80t
　supportive psychotherapy for, 80
Desipramine
　for anxiety, 71t
　for depression, 82t
　for neuropathic pain, 104
Developmental tasks of the dying, 15
Dexamethasone
　for anorexia-cachexia syndrome, 51t
　for bowel obstruction, 59t
　for cord compression, 127
　for fatigue, 84t
　for hematologic tumors, 119
　for increased intracranial pressure, 130
　for nausea management, 68t
Dexmethylphenidate, for fatigue, 84t
Dextroamphetamine
　for depression, 80t
　for fatigue, 84t
Dextromethorphan
　for chronic cough, 109
　for pain management, 102
Diarrhea, 59–61
　background information, 59
　chemotherapy-induced, 61
　evaluation
　　acute, 59
　　chronic, 60
　management, 60–61
　radiation-induced, 61
Diazepam
　for anxiety, 71t
　for nausea management, 68t
Diclofenac, for pain management, 91t
Diclofenac patch/cream/gel, for neuropathic pain, 105
Dilantin, for neuropathic pain, 104

Dimenhydrinate, for nausea
    management, 67t
Diphenhydramine
    for insomnia, 86t
    for nausea management, 67t
    for pruritus, 119
Diphenoxylate/atropine,
    for diarrhea, 60
Diuretics, for dyspnea, 111
Docusate calcium (kaopectate),
    for constipation, 57t
Docusate sodium,
    for constipation, 57t
Dolasetron, for nausea
    management, 67t
Donepezil, for fatigue, 84t
Dopamine antagonists, for nausea
    management, 67t
Doxepin
    for anxiety, 71t
    for depression, 82t
    for insomnia, 86t
    for neuropathic pain, 103
Doxepin cream, for neuropathic
    pain, 105
Dramamine, for nausea
    management, 67t
Dronabinol
    for anorexia-cachexia
      syndrome, 51t
    for nausea management, 68t
Droperidol, for nausea
    management, 67t
Dry mouth
    background information,
      62–63
    management, 64–65
Dry skin, 119
Duloxetine
    for depression, 81t
    for neuropathic pain, 104
Dyspepsia
    background information and
      evaluation, 61
    management of, 61–62
Dysphagia
    background information, 62

    evaluation, 63
    management, 63
Dyspnea
    background information and
      evaluation, 110
    management, 110–111
Dysuria, management, 54

E

Eastern Cooperative Oncology
    Group (ECOG), 31
Eicosapentaenoic acid, for
    anorexia-cachexia
    syndrome, 51t
Emend, for nausea
    management, 68t
Emergencies, 123–133
    actively dying, 123–124
    acute bleeding, 124–125
    anaphylaxis, 126
    cardiac tamponade, 126
    cord compression, 127
    hypercalcemia, 128–129
    increased intracranial pressure,
      129–130
    serotonin syndrome,
      130–131
    superior vena cava
      syndrome, 131
    tumor lysis syndrome, 132
    withdrawal syndromes, 133t
Emesis (vomiting). See Nausea and
    vomiting
EMLA cream
    for neuropathic pain, 105
    for pruritus, 119
Emotional suffering, ethical
    decision making and, 23
Empathic strategies, 14t
    empathic presence, 15
    empathic silence, 13
End-of-dose failure, pain and, 89
End-stage chronic kidney disease,
    pain management
    and, 107
End-stage liver disease, prognosis
    guidelines, 37

End-stage renal disease, prognosis
 guidelines, 38
Enemas, 58*t*
Epidural, for pain management, 106
Epinephrine
 for anaphylaxis, 126
 for bleeding from malodorous
  fungating wounds, 116
Episcopalians, views of suffering
 and dying by, 41*t*
Escitalopram
 for anxiety, 71*t*
 for depression, 81*t*
Estazolam, for insomnia, 85*t*
Eszopiclone, for insomnia, 85*t*
Ethical decision making, 23–30
Ethical principles, 23
Ethics consultation, 24–26
 approaches, 24–25
 goals, 24
 guidelines, 24
 models, 25
 performing, 26
 protocol for, 25–26
Ethnic views of suffering and dying,
 39*t*–40*t*
Etodolac, for pain management, 91*t*
Europeans, views of suffering and
 dying by, 39*t*
Euthanasia, physician-assisted, 30
Exercise, for pain
 management, 108
Exhaustion, palliative care team
 and, 12
Existential healing, 23
Extubation protocols,
 terminal, background
 information, evaluation,
 management, 114

F
FACT Spiritual History
 Assessment, 45*t*
Faith
 FACT Spiritual History
  Assessment, 45*t*
 spiritual history, 44

Famciclovir, for HSV, 64
Family communication, 18–21
 conflicts, 21
 "Dad's a fighter," 20
 "don't tell my mom," 20
 enhanced autonomy, 18
 family meeting, 18–19
 family systems theory, 18
 "I want you to do everything," 20
 refusal to participate or talk, 20
 SPIKES mnemonic, 19
 summary, 21
 "we are waiting for a
  miracle," 20
Famotidine, for dyspepsia and
 GERD, 61
FAST (Functional Assessment
 Stage), 32*t*
Fatigue
 background information,
  evaluation,
  management, 83
 pharmacologic interventions
  for, 84*t*
Fentanyl
 equianalgesic & pharmacokinetic
  table, 162*t*
 prescribing tips, 92, 95–96
Fentanyl IV, prescribing tips, 97
Fentanyl transdermal patch, for
 chronic pain, prescribing
 tips, 97
Fentora, 95
Filipinos, views of suffering and
 dying by, 40*t*
Fish oils, for fatigue, 84*t*
Fluconazole, for candidiasis, 64
Fluoxetine
 for anxiety, 71*t*
 for depression, 81*t*
Fluoxymesterone, for anorexia-
 cachexia syndrome, 50*t*
Flurazepam, for insomnia, 85*t*
Forming phase, collaborative team
 development, 11
Fresh frozen plasma, for acute
 bleeding, 125

Fungating wounds, malodorous, background information, evaluation, management, 115–116

G
Gabapentin
  for hiccups, 112
  for neuropathic pain, 104
  for neuropathic pruritus, 120
Gallium nitrate, for hypercalcemia, 129
Gastroesophageal reflux disease (GERD)
  background information and evaluation, 61
  management of, 61–62
Ghrelin/ghrelin analogues, 50*t*
Glucocorticoids, inhaled, for chronic cough, 109
Glycerin, for constipation, 57*t*
Glycopyrrolate
  for bowel obstruction, 59*t*
  for oral secretions, 113
  for urinary retention or overflow incontinence, 55
Goal setting, for patient, 15–16
Granisetron, for nausea management, 68*t*
Grief and bereavement, 75–79
  background information, 75
  evaluation, 77
  grief models, 77*t*
  managing grief for different groups, 78*t*–79*t*
  reactions to loss by age group, 76*t*
  writing condolence card, 79
Gum, sugar-free, for xerostomia, 64

H
H. pylori testing, 62
Halitosis
  background information, 63
  management, 65
Hallucinations, delirium and, 72

Haloperidol
  for anxiety, 71*t*
  for bowel obstruction, 59*t*
  for delirium, 74*t*
  for hiccups, 112
  for nausea management, 67*t*
Healthcare professionals, grief management for, 79*t*
Heart disease, hospice criteria, 33*t*
Heart failure, prognosis guidelines, 37
Hepatorenal syndrome, severe, prognosis guidelines for, 37
Hiccups
  background information, 111–112
  evaluation and management, 112
Hindus, views of suffering and dying by, 42*t*
HIV/AIDS, hospice criteria, 33*t*
Honey, for mucositis, 64
Hope, 15, 16
Hospice, 3
  basic services, 5*t*
  core and noncore services, 5
  criteria, 32*t*–34*t*
    prognostication guidelines, 31–32
  demographics, 9
  diagnosis, 9
  location, 8
  statistics, U.S., 2010, 8–9
  as subset of palliative care, 4
  whole person care, 5–6
HSV, management, 64
Hydration
  artificial, 51*t*
  diarrhea and, 60
Hydrocodone, equianalgesic & pharmacokinetic table, 162*t*
Hydromorphone
  dosages, 94
  equianalgesic & pharmacokinetic table, 162*t*
  prescribing tips, 92

Hydroxyzine, for nausea
    management, 67*t*
Hyoscyamine, for oral
    secretions, 113
Hyperalgesia, opioids and, 100
Hypercalcemia
    background information and
        evaluation, 128
    management, 128–129
Hypochondria, 69*t*

I

Ibuprofen, for pain
    management, 91*t*
Idiopathic pain, 89
Imipramine
    for anxiety, 71*t*
    for depression, 82*t*
    for insomnia, 86*t*
    for neuropathic pain, 103
Imodium, for diarrhea, 60
Inapsine, for nausea
    management, 67*t*
Incident pain, 89
Incontinence, 53
    management overview, 54*t*
    types of, 53
Indomethacin, for pain
    management, 91*t*
Infants
    hydromorphone dosages, 94
    morphine dosages, 94
Informed consent, 28
Insomnia
    background information,
        evaluation,
        management, 85
    pharmacologic therapy for,
        85*t*–86*t*
Intensive care unit, 35
Intracranial pressure (ICP),
    increased, 129–130
    background information, 129
    evaluation and management, 130
Intrathecal (subarachnoid), for
    pain management, side
    effects, 106

Ipratropium bromide, inhaled, for
    chronic cough, 109
Islam, views of suffering and dying
    in, 42*t*
Itching. *See* Pruritus

J

Jacobs stage theory of grief, 77*t*
Japanese, views of suffering and
    dying by, 40*t*
Jehovah's Witnesses, views of
    suffering and dying by, 42*t*
Judaism, views of suffering and
    dying in, 43*t*
Justice, clinical ethics, 23

K

Kadian, prescribing tips, 94
Kaopectate, 57*t*, 61
Karnofsky performance scale, 31
Kennedy terminal ulcer, 117
Ketamine
    for depression, 82*t*
    dosing, 102–103
    for pain management, side
        effects, 102
Ketoprofen, for pain
    management, 91*t*
Ketorolac, for pain
    management, 91*t*
Kidney disease, chronic, pain
    management and, 107
KPS. *See* Karnofsky performance
    scale
Kubler-Ross grief model, 77*t*
Kytril, for nausea management, 68*t*

L

Lactulose, for constipation, 57*t*
Lamictal, for neuropathic pain, 104
Lamotrigine, for neuropathic
    pain, 104
Law, physician-assisted suicide and
    euthanasia, 30
Lazanda, prescribing tips, 96
Lemon drops, for xerostomia, 64

Levorphanol, 94–95, 103
Lidocaine
  inhaled, for chronic cough, 109
  for neuropathic pain, 105
Lip balm, 64
Lithium, for depression, 82t
Liver disease
  end-stage, prognosis
    guidelines, 37
  hospice criteria, 33t
Lomotil, for diarrhea, 60
Loop diuretics, 128
Loperamide, for diarrhea, 60
Lorazepam
  for anxiety, 71t
  for delirium, 74t
  for insomnia, 85t
  for nausea management, 68t
Lubiprostone, for constipation, 57t
Lyrica, for neuropathic pain, 105

M
Maalox plus, for dyspepsia and
    GERD, 62
Magnesium hydroxide,
    for constipation, 57t
Malodorous fungating
    wounds, 115
Mannitol, for increased intracranial
    pressure, 130
Massage therapy, 70, 108
Meaning, universal search for, 15
Meclizine, for nausea
    management, 67t
Meclofenamate, for pain
    management, 92t
Medicine, goals of, 3
Meditation, pain management
    and, 108
Megace, for fatigue, 84t
Megestrol acetate, for anorexia-
    cachexia syndrome, 51t
Melatonin, for insomnia, 86t
MELD. See Model for end-stage liver
    disease
Meloxicam, for pain
    management, 92t

Meperidine, equianalgesic &
    pharmacokinetic
    table, 162t
Metastatic cancer, prognosis
    and, 31
Methadone
  equianalgesic & pharmacokinetic
    table, 163t
  for pain management, 102
  prescribing tips, 98
Methocarbamol, for pain
    management, 104
Methylphenidate
  for delirium, 74t
  for depression, 80t
  for fatigue, 84t
Metoclopramide
  for constipation, 58t
  for hiccups, 112
  for nausea management, 67t
Mexicans, views of suffering and
    dying by, 40t
Midazolam, for refractory symptoms
    of delirium, 75t
Middle Easterners, views of
    suffering and dying by, 39t
Midodrine
  for ascites, 52
  for fatigue, 84t
Milk of magnesium,
    for constipation, 57t
Mineral oil, for constipation, 57t
Mirtazapine
  for anxiety, 72t
  for depression, 81t
  for hematologic tumors, 119
  for insomnia, 86t
  for uremia, 120
Misoprostol, for dyspepsia and
    GERD, 62
Modafinil
  for depression, 80t
  for fatigue, 84t
Model for end-stage liver
    disease, 37
Mormons, views of suffering and
    dying by, 43t

Morphine, 106
  for chronic cough, 109
  dosages, 94
  for dyspnea, 111
  equianalgesic & pharmacokinetic
    table, 163t
  prescribing tips, 92
  for wound pain, 115
Mourning, 75
Mouthwash mixture,
  for mucositis, 64
Mucositis
  background information, 62
  grading, 63
  management, 64
Muscle relaxants
  for pain management, 104
  for urinary retention or overflow
    incontinence, 55
Music therapy, for pain
  management, 108
Myoclonus, opioids and, 100

N
Nabumetone, for pain
  management, 92t
Naloxone
  for cholestasis, 120
  for constipation, 58t
  overdose, 101
Naltrexone, for uremia, 119
Naproxen, for pain
  management, 91t
Nasal cannula, 114
Native Americans, views of
  suffering and dying by, 39t
Nausea and vomiting
  background information, 65–66
  evaluation, 66
  management, 66
  medications for, 67t–68t
  opioids and, 100
Neonates, morphine dosages, 94
Nerve blocks, side effects, 106
Neurokinin 1 antatonists,
  for nausea management, 68t
Neuroleptics, for anxiety, 71t

Neurological diseases, hospice
  criteria, 34t
Neuropathic pain
  description, 87–88
  managing, 103–104
Neuropsychiatric, 69–86
  anxiety, 69–72
  delirium, 72–75
  depression, 79–83
  fatigue, 84
  grief and bereavement, 75–79
  insomnia, 85, 85t–86t
Nitrates, for heart failure, 111
NMDA antagonists, for pain
  management, 102–105
Nociceptive pain, somatic or
  visceral, 87
Nonmaleficence, clinical ethics, 23
Non-opioid analgesics, for pain
  management, 90t–92t
Norming phase, collaborative team
  development and, 11
Nortriptyline
  for anxiety, 71t
  for depression, 82t
  for neuropathic pain, 103
NSAIDs
  for pain management, 89–90
  for pruritus, 119
  for tumor-related pruritus, 119
NURSE mnemonic, 18
Nursing home patients, Porock
  6-month risk calculation
  for, 38
Nutrition, artificial, 51t

O
Obsessive-compulsive disorder, 69t
Octreotide
  for acute bleeding, 125
  for bowel obstruction, 59t
  for chemotherapy-induced
    diarrhea, 61
Olanzapine
  for anxiety, 71t
  for delirium, 74t
  for nausea management, 67t

Omega-3 fatty acids, for
fatigue, 84*t*
Ondansetron
for hematologic tumors, 119
for nausea management, 68*t*
Onsolis, prescribing tips, 96
Opiates, for diarrhea, 60
Opioid antagonists,
for constipation, 58*t*
Opioids
addiction, 101
for chronic cough, 109
converting from oral methadone
to oral morphine, 99
converting to IV methadone,
99–100
for cord compression, 127
for dyspnea, 111
equianalgesic & pharmacokinetic
table, 162*t*–163*t*
overdose, 100–101
prescribing tips, 92
pseudoaddiction, 101–102
side effects, managing,
100–102
for terminal extubation
protocols, 114
for urinary retention or overflow
incontinence, 55
withdrawal syndromes, 133*t*
Opium, for bladder or ureteral
spasms, 54–55
Oral hygiene, for halitosis, 65
Oral secretions
background information, 112
evaluation, 112
management, 113
Oropharynx, care, 62–65
Overflow incontinence, 53–54, 55
Oxandrolone, 50*t*
Oxazepam, for anxiety, 71*t*
Oxcarbazepine, for neuropathic
pain, 104
Oxybutynin
for urinary retention or overflow
incontinence, 55
for urinary symptoms, 54

Oxycodone
equianalgesic & pharmacokinetic
table, 163*t*
prescribing tips, 92, 95
Oxygen, for dyspnea, 111
Oxymorphone
equianalgesic & pharmacokinetic
table, 163*t*
prescribing tips, 95

P
Packed red blood cells, for acute
bleeding, 125
Pain, 87–108
assessment, 88
background information, 87
breakthrough, 89
chronic kidney disease, 107
cirrhosis, 107
complementary
therapies, 108
documenting
adults, 88
children, 88–89
management, 89–108
anesthetics, 105
anticonvulsant medications,
104–105
antidepressants,
103–104
antispasmodics/muscle
relaxants, 104
bisphosphonates/osteoclast
inhibitors, 103
cannabinoids, 105
corticosteroids, 103
NMDA antagonists,
102–103
non-opioid analgesics,
90*t*–92*t*
NSAIDs, 89–90
opioids, 92–102
steps, 89
topical agents, 105
WHO ladder, 89
neuropathic, 87–88
nociceptive, 87

procedures, 106
radiopharmaceutical therapies, 106–107
visceral, 107
Pain assessment tool, *164*
PAIN mnemonic, 87
Pain sensation scale, *165*
Palliative care
goal of, 3
pediatrics and, 7
principles of, 4
Palliative care teams, 11–12
burnout/burnout-reduction techniques, 12
clinical ethics, 23
collaborative team development phases, 11–12
forming, 11
norming, 11
performing, 11
storming, 11
conflicts, 12
effectiveness of, 12
team model and composition, 11
Palliative performance scale, 31
Palliative prognostic index, 31
Palliative prognostic score, 31
Palonosetron, for nausea management, 68*t*
Pamidronate
for hypercalcemia, 129
pain management and, 103
Panic disorder, 69*t*
PaP. *See Palliative prognostic score*
Parental support, pediatrics and, 7
Paroxetine
for anxiety, 71*t*
for depression, 81*t*
for hematologic tumors, 119
for polycythemia vera, 120
Patient communication
barriers to, 13–14
basics, 13
elements of, 13
empathic strategies, 14*t*
goal setting, 15–16

Patient-controlled analgesia (PCA), 93
Pediatrics
palliative care and, 7
parental support, 7
Pentobarbital, for terminal anxiety/agitation, 72*t*
Performing phase, collaborative team development and, 11
Pet therapy, 70
Phenazopyridine, for urinary symptoms, 54
Phenergan, for nausea management, 67*t*
Phenobarbital
for refractory symptoms of delirium, 75*t*
for terminal anxiety/agitation, 72*t*
Phenytoin
for hiccups, 112
for neuropathic pain, 104
Phototherapy, for uremia, 119
Physician-assisted suicide and euthanasia, 30
Pilocarpine, for dry mouth, 65
Pimecrolimus 1% cream, for pruritus, 119
Piroxicam, for pain management, 92*t*
Platelet transfusions, for acute bleeding, 125
Pleural effusions, background information, evaluation, management, 113
Pleurodesis options, 113
Polyethylene glycol, for constipation, 57*t*
Porock 6-month risk, calculating, 38
Positioning, for dyspnea, 111
PPI. *See Palliative prognostic index*
PPS. *See Palliative performance scale*
Pramipexole, for insomnia, 86*t*
Pramoxine, for pruritus, 119
Prayer, pain management and, 108
Prednisone, for fatigue, 84*t*

Pregabalin
  for neuropathic pain, 105
  for neuropathic pruritus, 120
Pressure ulcers
  background information and
    evaluation, 117
  management, 118
Probiotics, for diarrhea, 61
Prochlorperazine maleate, for
    nausea management, 67t
Prognosis, reviewing, 19
Prognostication, 31–38
  ADO Index, 36t–37t
  basic information, 31–32
  Child-Pugh class, 38t
  guidelines by disease
    cancer, 35
    chronic obstructive lung
      disease, 36
    dementia, 38
    end-stage liver disease, 37
    end-stage renal disease, 38
    heart failure, 37
  hospice criteria, 32t–34t
Progressive muscle relaxation, for
    anxiety, 70
Progestins, for anorexia-cachexia
    syndrome, 51t
Prokinetics
  for anorexia-cachexia
    syndrome, 51t
  for constipation, 58t
  for dyspepsia and GERD, 62
  for nausea management, 67t
Promethazine, for nausea
    management, 67t
Propofol
  for refractory symptoms of
    delirium, 75t
  for terminal anxiety/
    agitation, 72t
Propranolol, for anxiety, 72t
Protestants, views of suffering and
    dying by, 43t
Provigil, for fatigue, 84t
Prune juice, for constipation, 57t

Pruritus (itching), 118–120
  background information, 118
  evaluation, 118–119
  management, 119–120
  opioids and, 101
Pulmonary diseases, hospice
    criteria, 33t
PUVA, for polycythemia vera, 120

Q

Quality of life, ethics consultation
    and, 26
Quetiapine
  for anxiety, 71t
  for delirium, 74t

R

Radiopharmaceutical therapies,
    for pain management,
    106–107
Ramelteon, for insomnia, 86t
Ranitidine, for dyspepsia and
    GERD, 61
Rasburicase, for tumor lysis
    syndrome, 132
Reglan, for nausea
    management, 67t
Relationship building, 15
Relaxation therapy
  for anxiety, 70
  for dyspnea, 111
Religious views of suffering and
    dying, 41t–43t
REMS, transmucosal fentanyl
    products and, 95
Renal failure, hospice criteria, 34t
Resource allocation, ethics
    consultation and, 25
Respiratory, 109–114
  chronic cough, 109
  dyspnea, 110–111
  hiccups, 111–112
  oral secretions, 112–113
  pleural effusions, 113
  terminal extubation
    protocols, 114

Respiratory depression, opioids and, 101
Risk evaluation and mitigation strategy. See REMS
Risperidone
 for anxiety, 71t
 for delirium, 74t
Russians, views of suffering and dying by, 40t

S
SAAG, calculating, 52
Saliva substitutes, 64
Salsalate, for pain management, 90t
Scopolamine
 for nausea management, 67t
 for oral secretions, 113
 for urinary retention or overflow incontinence, 55
Selective serotonin reuptake inhibitors
 for anxiety, 70, 71t
 for depression, 81t
 withdrawal syndromes, 133t
Self-disclosure, limiting, 18
Senna, for constipation, 57t
Separation-anxiety disorder, 69t
Serotonin 5HT3 antagonists, for nausea management, 67t–68t
Serotonin syndrome
 background information and evaluation, 130
 management, 131
Sertraline
 for anxiety, 71t
 for depression, 81t
Shared decision making, 27–28
 decisional capacity assessment, 27
 informed consent, 28
 legal concerns, 27–28
Sikh, views of suffering and dying by, 43t

Silence, empathic, 13
Silver nitrate, for bleeding from malodorous fungating wounds, 116
Simethicone, for abdominal bloating and gas, 55
Skin, 115–120
 malodorous fungating wounds, 115–116
 pressure ulcers, 117–118
 pruritus, 118–120
Social phobia, 69t
Social services, 11
Somatic pain, 87
South Asians, views of suffering and dying by, 40t
SPIKES mnemonic, 17, 19
Spinal cord compression, 127
Spiritual assessment, 44
Spiritual counselor, 11
Spiritual history and interventions, 44
Spiritual screen, 44
Spiritual views of suffering and dying, 41t–43t
SSRIs. See Selective serotonin reuptake inhibitors
Steroids, for nausea management, 68t
Stool softeners, 57t
Storming phase, collaborative team development and, 11
Stress, palliative care team and, 12
Stress incontinence, 53
Stretching, for pain management, 108
Stroke, hospice criteria, 34t
Sucralfate, for dyspepsia and GERD, 62
Suffering, 87
 ethical decision making and, 23
 ethnic views of, 39t–40t
 religious views of, 41t–43t
Suicide, physician-assisted, 30
Sulindac, for pain management, 91t

Superior vena cava (SVC) syndrome, background information, evaluation, management, 131

Surrogates, legally identified, 28

T

Tacrolimus ointment, for pruritus, 119

Temazepam
  for anxiety, 71*t*
  for insomnia, 85*t*

Terminal patients, ED visit diagnosis reasons, 6*t*

Testosterone, for fatigue, 84*t*

Thalidomide
  for anorexia-cachexia syndrome, 51*t*
  for chronic cough, 109
  for fatigue, 84*t*
  for uremia, 119

Theophylline, for dyspnea, 111

Thiopental, for terminal anxiety/agitation, 72*t*

Thoracentesis, for pleural effusions, 113

Thorazine, for nausea management, 67*t*

Thromboplastin, for bleeding from malodorous fungating wounds, 116

Tigan, for nausea management, 68*t*

Tizanidine, for pain management, 104

Tolterodine, for urinary symptoms, 54

Topical agents, for neuropathic pain, 105

Topiramate, for neuropathic pain, 105

Toradol, for pain management, 91*t*

Tramadol
  equianalgesic & pharmacokinetic table, 163*t*
  prescribing tips, 100

Tranexamic acid, for acute bleeding, 125

Trazodone
  for depression, 81*t*
  for insomnia, 86*t*
  for neuropathic pain, 104

Treatment, withholding *vs.* withdrawing, 28–29

Triazolam, for insomnia, 85*t*

Tricyclic antidepressants
  for anxiety, 71*t*
  for depression, 82*t*

Trigger-point injections, 106

Triiodothyronine, for depression, 82*t*

Trileptal, for neuropathic pain, 104

Trimethobenzamide, for nausea management, 68*t*

Tumor lysis syndrome, background information, evaluation, management, 132

U

Ulcers, pressure, 117–118

Uncomplicated (normal) grief, 76

Understanding, 13

Uremia, 119

Ureteral spasms, management, 54–55

Urge incontinence, 53

Urinary retention, management, 55

Urinary symptoms, 53–55
  evaluation, 53
  management, 54–55

V

Valacyclovir, for HSV, 64

Valproate, for neuropathic pain, 105

Valsalva technique, for hiccups, 112

Venlafaxine
  for depression, 81*t*
  for neuropathic pain, 104

Venlafaxine XR, for anxiety, 72*t*
Vietnamese, views of suffering and
    dying by, 40*t*
Visceral pain, 87, 107
Vitamin K, for acute bleeding, 125
Vocabulary barriers, 14
Volunteers, 11
Vomiting. *See* Nausea and vomiting
Vomiting center, 65

W
WHO ladder, pain management
    and, 89
Whole person care, 5–6
Withdrawal syndromes, 133*t*
Withholding *vs.* withdrawing
    treatment, 28–29
Wounds, malodorous fungating, 115

X
Xerosis (dry skin), 118
Xerostomia (dry mouth)
    background information,
        62–63
    management, 64–65
Xylocaine, for mucositis, 64

Z
Zaleplon, for insomnia, 85*t*
Ziconotide, 106
Zofran, for nausea
    management, 68*t*
Zoledronic acid
    for hypercalcemia, 129
    pain management
        and, 103
Zolpidem, for insomnia, 85*t*

Opioid Equianalgesic & Pharmacokinetic Table

Current Opioid/24 h × (New Opioid/24 h × (New Opioid Factor/Current Opioid Route Factor) = New Opioid/24 h

Drug	IV (mg)	PO (mg)	Onset	Peak (prn = 10% of daily)	Duration	Half-life (for routine dosing)	Comments: For incomplete cross-tolerance adjustment (except fentanyl & methadone): pain 7–10, no adjustment; 4–6, 25% reduction; 1–3, 50% reduction.
Buprenorphine SL: 2, 8 mg. TD: 5, 10, 20 mg	0.3	0.4 (SL)	10–30 min (IM)	60 m (IM)	6–8 h (IV)	2–3 h (IV)	Sublingual tablets (Subutex) and transdermal patches (Butrans) available (for mod pain). Schedule III like Vicodin and Tyl w/codeine.
Codeine	130	200	30–60 min	1–2 h (PO)	4–6 h	3 h	Weak opioid. Prodrug, metabolized to morphine in the liver. 10% nonresponders. Tylenol #3 = 30 mg #4 = 60 mg.
Fentanyl Dermal: 12, 25, 50, 75, 100 mcg Lozenge: 200, 400, 600, 800, 1200, 1600 mcg Buccal: 100, 200, 400, 600, 800 mcg	100 mcg (acute); see comments	n/a	1 min (IV) 5–15 min (lozenge) 12 h (patch)	36 h (patch) 20–60 min (lozenge) 6–15 min (IV)	48–72 h (patch) 1 h (lozenge) 2 h (buccal) 30–60 min (IV)	13–22 h (patch) 7 h (lozenge) 2–12 h (buccal)	PREFERRED IN RENAL OR HEPATIC FAILURE. Steady state can take up to 36 h 1 mcg/h transdermal = 2 mg/24 h morphine PO (takes into account crosstolerance). Example: 25 mcg/h fentanyl patch chronic dosing = approx 50 mg/24 h of morphine PO (or approx 1 mg/h morphine IV) If patch removed: half eliminated in 17 h.
Hydrocodone	n/a	30	10–20 min	1–2 h	4–6 h	4 h	Consider with caution in hepatic dysfunction. Combination products (Vicodin, Lorcet 10 mg, Lortab 5/7.5/10 mg, Norco 5/7.5/10 mg, Vicoprofen 7.5 mg). CAUTION: total acetaminophen dose.
Hydromorphone PO: 2, 4, 8, 1 mg/mL PR: 3 mg ER: 8, 12, 16 mg	1.5	7.5	30 min (PO) 5 min (IV)	60 min (PO) 15 min (IV) 30 min (SQ)	4–5 h (IR)	2–3 h (IR)	Consider with caution in renal or hepatic dysfunction (using reduced dosing and intervals). Some studies imply oral equianalgesic dose likely closer to 3.
Meperidine PO: 50, 100, 10 mg/mL	100	300	5 min (IV) 10 min (PO)	30–60 min (PO)	2–3 h (PO)	20 h metabolite	NOT RECOMMENDED for clinical use, if must use then limit to <48 h with reduced dosing.

	24 h oral dose / 2 = 24 h IV dose; (from IV back to oral = x1.3)	See comments	10–120 min (PO) 10–20 min (IV)	2–4 h (PO) –1 h (IV)	6–12 h	15–190 h (≥3 h)	PREFERRED IN RENAL FAILURE. Steady state in 4–10 days.
Methadone PO: 5, 10, 5 mg/mL, 10 mg, 10 mg/mL: mg only for substance abuse centers)							24 oral morphine dose: <100 (3.1:) 101–300 (5.1:) 301–600 (10:1) 601–800 (12:1) 801–1000 (15:1) / >1000 (20:1) Decrease result by 50% (multiply by 0.5) –75% (multiply by 0.25) Example: 195 mg oral morphine/5 = 39/day = ×0.5 or ×0.25 = 9.8 to 19.5/day methadone
Morphine IR: 15, 30 tabs; 10 mg/5 mL, 20 mg/5 mL, 100 mg/5 mL; SR: 15, 30, 60, 100, 200 mg; PR: 5, 10, 20, 30 mg	10	30	30 min (PO) 5–10 min (IV)	1 h (IR) 4 h (SR) 10 min (IV)	3–4 h (IR) 8–12 h (SR)	1.5–2 h (4 h including active metabolites) (IR)	Consider with caution with hepatic dysfunction. With chronic dosing, oral equivalent is closer to 20. Metabolized to morphine –3 & 6-glucomide –> M6G is active and has a 4 h half-life (accumulates in renal failure, reduce dosage). Note: extended-release Avinza peaks in 30 minutes, Kadian in 9 h.
Oxycodone PO: 5, 10, 15, 20, 30, 5 mg/ 5 mL, 20 mg/ml SR: 10, 15, 20, 30, 40, 60, 80	n/a	20	10–10 min (PO)	1–2 h (po)	3–4 h (IR) 8–12 h (SR)	3–4 h (IR) 4.5–8 h (SR)	Consider with caution in hepatic dysfunction. Available alone (OxyFast, OxyIR, OxyContin) or combination (Endocet 5/7.5/10, Percocet 2.5/5/7.5/10, Roxicet 5). CAUTION: total acetaminophen dose.
Oxymorphone IR: 5, 10 mg ER: 5, 7.5, 10, 15, 20, 30, 40 mg	1	10	30 min (PO) 5–10 min (IV)	1–2 h	3–6 h	7–9 h (IR) 9–11 h (ER)	Opana. Delayed time to peak if taken with food. Alcohol can increase drug release from ER tablet. AVOID combination.
Tramadol IR/ODT: 50 mg ER: 100, 200, 300 mg	n/a	120	1 h (IR)	2 h (IR)	4–6 h	6–8 h	Ultram. Weak opioid. Active metabolite. Also has SNRI-like activity (avoid if MAOI use within 14 days).

Information from: 1) The 5th Vital Sign Chart (Updated May 2010, ViaHealth Pain Initiative, downloaded from http://www.compassionandsupport.org/pdfs/professionals/pain/equi_table_(EX).pdf June 20, 2012; 2) Lexi-Comp Online, Pediatric Lexi-Drugs Online, Hudson, Ohio: Lexi-Comp, Inc. 2012; June 20, 2012.); 3) Wu, Patty Patty WU's Palliative Medicine Pocket Consultation. San Diego, CA: The Institute for Palliative Medicine at San Diego Hospice, 2009 and 4) McPherson Mary L. Demystifying Opioid Conversion Calculations: A Guide for Effective Dosing. Bethesda, MD: American Society of Health-System Pharmacists. 2010.

	0	1	2	3	4	5	6	7	8	9	10
Verbal descriptive scale	No pain		Mild pain		Moderate pain		Moderate pain		Severe pain		Worst pain possible
	Alert smiling		No humor Serious Flat		Furrowed brow Pursed lips Breath holding		Wrinkled nose Raised upper lip Rapid breathing		Slow blink Open mouth		Eyes closed Moaning Crying
Activity tolerance scale	No pain		Can be ignored		Interferes with tasks		Interferes with concentration		Interferes with basic needs		Bedrest required

This pain assessment tool is intended to help patient care providers assess pain according to individual patient needs. Explain and use 0-10 scale for patient self-assessment. Use the faces or behavioral observations to interpret expressed pain when patient cannot communicate his/her pain intensity.

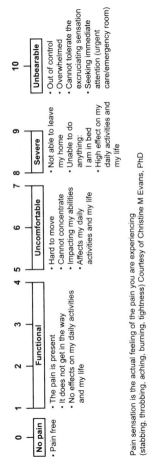

	0	1	2	3	4	5	6	7	8	9	10

No pain
- Pain free

Functional
- The pain is present
- It does not get in the way
- No effects on my daily activities and my life

Uncomfortable
- Hard to move
- Cannot concentrate
- Impacting my abilities
- Affects my daily activities and my life

Severe
- Not able to leave my home
- Unable to do anything: I am in bed
- High effect on my daily activities and my life

Unbearable
- Out of control
- Overwhelmed
- Cannot tolerate the excruciating sensation
- Seeking immediate attention (urgent care/emergency room)

Pain sensation is the actual feeling of the pain you are experiencing (stabbing, throbbing, aching, burning, tightness) Courtesy of Christine M Evans, PhD